Yousra Fakhfakh
Imen Frikha

Diagnosis and treatment of acute lymphoblastic leukemia

Yousra Fakhfakh
Imen Frikha

Diagnosis and treatment of acute lymphoblastic leukemia

ScienciaScripts

Cover image: www.ingimage.com

This book is a translation from the original published under ISBN 978-620-6-72203-8.

Publisher:
Sciencia Scripts
is a trademark of
Dodo Books Indian Ocean Ltd. and OmniScriptum S.R.L publishing group

120 High Road, East Finchley, London, N2 9ED, United Kingdom
Str. Armeneasca 28/1, office 1, Chisinau MD-2012, Republic of Moldova, Europe
Printed at: see last page
ISBN: 978-620-8-18490-2

Contents

Dedication

All the letters can't find the right words...
All the words can
't express gratitude, love,
respect, gratitude...
So it's quite simply that

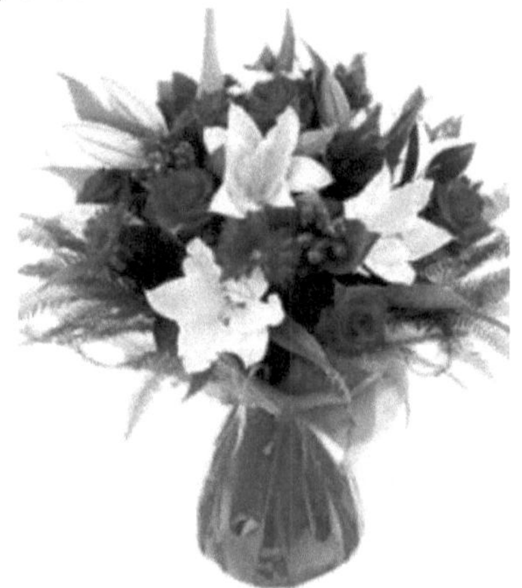

I dedicate this thesis.

TO MY VERY DEAR FATHER :
ABDELJALIL

Gt _S>

To the person who helped me discover the inexhaustible treasure of 'savoi'.
Of all the people I've loved, you've been the best,
instilled in me the noble values of life, taught me the meaning of work,
honesty and responsibility.
Thank you for always being there for me, a great support throughout my
studies.
my studies. You were and always will be an example to follow for your
human
human qualities, your perseverance and your perfectionism.
Words can never express the depth of my respect,
consideration, gratitude and eternal love.
This work is your work, you who have given me so much and you
continue to do so... without ever complaining.
I wish I could return all the love and devotion you have given us
but a lifetime would not be enough. I hope that this
work will at least contribute to
that.

TO MY VERY DEAR MOTHER:
SONIA

So many sentences, no matter how expressive, cannot show the degree of
degree of love and affection I feel for you.
You have filled me with your tenderness and affection throughout my
journey.
journey.
You never ceased to support and encourage me throughout my years
of study, and you were always there to comfort me when I needed it.
when I needed it.
On this memorable day, for myself as well as for you, let me present this
work as a
as a sign of my deep gratitude and esteem.
May the Almighty give you health, happiness and long life so that
so that I can fill you in my turn.

A Mon PETIT
YOUSSEF

All the letters can't find the right words...
No words can express love....
In short, you are the joy of my life. I hope that my thesis will be
a source of pride for you and an example to follow.
Your zest for life and your smile have been the best encouragement
encouragement I could ever have.
May God watch over you and protect you.

To My DEARJEPOUX
MOHAMMED AYMEN

Your encouragement and support were the breath of fresh air that
revitalised me
in times of pain, loneliness and suffering.
Thank you for always being by my side, with your presence, your love
and tenderness, to give flavour and meaning to our family life.
family life.
As a token of my love, admiration and great
affection, please find in this work the expression of my esteem
and my sincere attachment.
I pray to Almighty God to give you happiness and prosperity.

A MA CHERE SOUR
YOLDES AND HER HUSBAND AHMED

Those who have shared my joys and sufferings with me
Those who fill me with their love and tenderness
May this work be an expression of my eternal and sincere fraternity,
of my great love and of my attachment to you.
May god keep us united and happy and grant us health, happiness
and success

.

TO MY BROTHER
YESSINE

Tugardes always has a special place in my heart
May you find in this work the testimony of my love and dedication
attachment
I wish you much happiness and good health

TO MY MOTHER-IN-LAW
TATA FATHIA

I could never express the respect I have for you.
Your prayers, encouragement and support have always been
a great help to me

.

May Almighty God preserve you from evil, fill you with health
health and happiness
and give you a long life.

IN MEMORY OF MY FATHER-IN-LAW
TOUAFIK

I wish you could have been there.
May your soul rest in peace and may God offer you Paradise as your
eternal
resting place.

TO MY GRANDMOTHER
SOUAD

You have always supported and encouraged me.
This is the day you've been waiting for more impatiently than I have, and it
will be
an opportunity to share the joy.
It gives me great pleasure to dedicate this modest work to you.
May God bring you health and happiness.

IN MEMORY OF MY GRAND PARENTS
AMEUR, SADOK and LATIFA

I miss you very much.
May your souls rest in peace and may God shower you with grace.

IN MEMORY OF MY TENT FADOUA

I really miss you.
Absent today, you are always present in our conversations.
You were always there to listen to me.
I would have loved loved having you there.
May god bless your soul and offer you paradise as your eternal resting
place.
eternal rest.

TO MY BROTHER-IN-LAW NIZAR, HIS WIFE ABIR
AND THEIR SON TAOUFIK

As a token of my deep attachment
and gratitude for all your help and support
May God keep us united and grant us health, happiness and success.

TO MY BEAUTIFUL SO.URLOBNA, HER HUSBAND MOHAMMED AND THEIR SONS MOHAMMED, MAHDI AND MALEK

May this work be the expression of a sincere and eternal fraternity, of my great love and attachment
May God keep us united and grant us health, happiness and success.

A

MY UNCLES AND THEIR WIVES

MY TENTS AND THEIR SPOUSES

ALL MY COUSINS

TO ALL THE FAMILY

FAKHFAKH

ZOUARI

DERBEL

Through this work, I express to you all the love and respect that I owe you.
I owe you.

TO MY DEAR FRIENDS

Asma koubaa and her husband Nizar and their sons Youssef,
Hela and her husband Ali and their daughter Mariem,
Sameh and her husband Slim and their daughter chahd,
Nihel and her husband Omar and their daughter Lina,
Wafa and her husband Mohammed and their children,
Ines and her husband and their children,
Rahma Mallek and her husband and their children.

TO MY DEAR FRIENDS

Abir Miled, Rachid Kharrat, Neder Slema, Nedia Ameur, Tarak ben Jmeaa, Imen Abdelli, Sana Ennouri, Syrine Sgaier, Abir Derbel, Zeineb Mlayah.

Acknowledgements

Our Master and President of the Jury
Dear Professor
MOEZ ELLOUMI
Head of the haematology department
at the Hedi Chafer University Hospital in Sfax
You are doing us a great honour by accepting the presidency.
of the jury for our thesis.
Your advice was invaluable in helping us to complete this project.
You have enriched us with your valuable teaching and
experience,
We have always admired and respected you,
your great modesty and your great human qualities
Your scientific rigour, professional awareness
and teaching skills have touched us deeply.
Please find in this modest work the expression of our
deep esteem and sincere gratitude.
Our Master and judge
Professor
Hdiji probes
Haematology department
at the Hedi Chaker University Hospital in Sfax.

You have done us the great honour of agreeing to judge these.
Your rich and in-depth knowledge, your vast experience
and your scientific rigour, will have a beneficial influence on each of your disciples.
on each and every one of your disciples.
During all the courses we were able to appreciate your exemplary qualities,
your human and professional qualities, your seriousness, your dedication and your
extreme kindness.
Please accept this letter as an expression of my respect and
gratitude.
Our Master and Judge
Professor *areg-*
Hela Mnif

Sfax Regional Blood Transfusion Centre
You have done us the great honour of agreeing to judge these.
Your extreme kindness and knowledge have always impressed us.
You have always inspired us with respect and admiration for your very high

human and professional qualities, your integrity and your quest for the best.

Our Master and Jugf Professor agregf

Moez Medhaffar

Fhematology Department

, CHU Hedi Chaker, Sfax.

You have done us the great honour of agreeing to judge these.

We were lucky enough to be among your students and to be able to benefit from your great knowledge. Your skill, your constant quest for perfection, your kindness and and your modesty are much admired.

In these few lines we would like to express our sincere gratitude and deep respect.

Please find in this work the testimony of our deep respect and our sincere gratitude.

Our Master and Judge

Professor *agregf*

Nour Abdeljlil

National marrow transplant centre

Bone of Tunis

By agreeing to judge this modest work, you are doing us the greatest honour.

Please find in this work, Dear Master, the expression of our great esteem and profound gratitude.

A

Our Master and director of these

Dear Doctor

Imen Frikha

Department of Hematology

, CHU Hedi Chaker - Sfax

You have done us a great honour in accepting the direction of this work and guiding us throughout.

Your advice and precious instructions, always given with the utmost friendliness have enabled us to develop this work.

Your patience, your modesty, your constant availability, your qualities respect and admiration.

Your tireless efforts to achieve ever-greater perfection have touched our hearts.

Please find herewith the testimony of our great respect, immense admiration and profound gratitude.

A

Professor Hatem Bellaaj

Professor Olfa Kasssar

Dr Manel Ghorbel

Dr Feten Kallel
Dr Maha Charfi
Dr Imen Ben Amor
A
All paramedical and medical staff
From the Sfax clinical haematology department
De carcinologie medicale de Sfax
Du centre regional de transfusion snaguine
May you find in these words my best wishes for happiness and success.

All My Masters
From the Sfax dermatology department
From the Sfax infectious diseases department
Sfax cardiovascular department Sfax obstetric gynecology
department Sfax neonatology
department Sfax radiology department
As well as
All the paramedical staff in these departments

Please find here Γ expression of my sincere respect

1 Introduction

Acute lymphoblastic leukaemia (ALL) is a clonal proliferation developed from a lymphoid cell blocked at an early stage of differentiation (1). The main consequences of this proliferation are the development of medullary insufficiency, which may be associated with febrile neutropenia, anemic syndrome and haemorrhagic syndrome, and the appearance of a tumour syndrome (2).

ALL is the most common cancer in children (3), although it is relatively rare in adults, with an incidence of 1 new case/100,000 inhabitants/year (4). Prognostic factors have been well defined, including t(9,22), which is the most frequent cytogenetic abnormality with a poor prognosis in adults. In fact, phi+ ALL represents 3% of childhood ALL and its incidence is constantly increasing, reaching 20-30% in adulthood and 50% from the age of 50.

The prognosis of adult ALL has improved considerably over the last 20 years, thanks to improved prognostic stratification and the use of new therapies tailored to prognostic factors (5,6). However, the prognosis remains guarded, with a prolonged survival probability of 30-40%, in contrast to childhood ALL, which has an overall five-year survival of 80-90% (5,6).

In our centre, the hematology department of the Hedi Chaker University Hospital in Sfax, the treatment of ALL was based on the administration of polychemotherapy according to the French protocols LALA 76, LALA 87 and HPS 89. An initial evaluation was carried out in 1999 in a study by *S. Nasf* (7), showing inadequate results compared with the various series in the literature, with a 5-year OS and 5-year follow-up of 14% and 12% respectively. With the aim of improving our results, the LALA 94 protocol was used from 1996 onwards, and an evaluation was carried out in 2003 as part of a multicentre study which still produced disappointing results, with an OS of around 20% (8). Since then, French therapeutic protocols inspired by paediatric protocols have been used, namely GRAALL/ GRAAPH 2003 and 2005.

Through a retrospective study of 49 cases of adult ALL followed at the hematology department of Sfax and treated according to a protocol inspired by GRAALL / GRAAPH during the period from 2004 to 2015, we study :

- Epidemiological, clinical and biological profile of ALL in southern Tunisia.
- The therapeutic results of these GRAALL / GRAAPH-inspired protocols during this period.
- Overall survival, event-free survival and relapse-free survival and determine the prognostic factors.
- To propose a new version of the treatment protocol for adult ALL in southern Tunisia.

2 Patient and methods

1 Patients

Our study is retrospective and concerned all patients aged between 20 and 56 years with de novo acute lymphoblastic leukaemia diagnosed in the hematology department of the Hedi Chaker University Hospital in Sfax and treated according to a protocol inspired by GRAALL / GRAAPH 2003 and 2005, over a 12-year period from January 2004 to December 2015.

2 Methods

A form has been designed to collect epidemiological, clinical, biological, therapeutic and evolutionary data.

2.1 Epidemiological data

For each patient, we specified age, sex, month and year of diagnosis, as well as governorate of origin.

2.2 Clinical data

We have looked for this in our patients:

- The presence of a tumour syndrome: adenopathies, splenomegaly, hepatomegaly.
- Damage to the central nervous system: clinical and/or biological.

CNS involvement is defined by the presence of cranial nerve palsies or other significant neurological involvement and/or the presence of leukemic cells in the cerebrospinal fluid and/or the presence of mononuclear cells greater than or equal to $5*10^6$ /l associated with blast cells on a centrifugal CSF sample (9).

- Testicular involvement: by clinical examination (+/- trans-illumination) and if there is any doubt about the diagnosis, a testicular ultrasound or MRI scan will be requested.
- Signs of medullary insufficiency: the anemic syndrome, the haemorrhagic syndrome and the infectious syndrome with the different possible foci.

2.3 Biological data

2.3.1 *Hemogram with blood smear*

Performed on all patients to determine the white blood cell (WBC)/mm^3 , the haemoglobin (Hb) in g/dL and the platelet count (Pq)/ mm^3 . The smear is taken after a drop of blood has been spread between the slide and the coverslip. After staining with the May-Grunwald-Giemsa stain, it is used to visualise blood infiltration by blasts and to describe their morphology. It is performed at the hematology laboratory of the Habib Bourguiba University Hospital in Sfax.

2.3.2 *Hemostasis assessment*

PT, aPTT, Fg and D-dimer to look for DIC.

2.3.3 *Biochemical balance*

Blood ionogram, lactate dehydrogenase (LDH) levels, urea, creatinine, uricemia, calcium and phosphorus levels to check for tumour lysis syndrome.

2.3.4 *Myelogram*

The myelogram was analysed in the hematology laboratory of the Habib Bourguiba University Hospital in Sfax, confirming the diagnosis of LA and showing blastic infiltration >20%. The lymphoid nature of the blasts was confirmed by the absence of cytoplasmic granulations and by cytoplasmic myeloperoxidase (MPO) activity in less than 3% of blasts.

2.3.5 ***Immunophenotyping of blast cells***

2.3.5.1 ***Flow cytometry***

The bone marrow or peripheral blood sample, in the event of difficult medullary aspiration, is collected in a tube with lithium heparinate and stored at room temperature.

Flow cytometry analysis was carried out systematically in different laboratories depending on the period: Institut Pasteur in Tunis, hematology laboratory at Aziza Othmana Hospital in Tunis and CRTS in Sfax.

The diagnosis of B or T ALL is determined according to the EGIL criteria (Table I).

Table I: EGIL classification of ALL.

Toutes les LAL B ont au moins 2 des 3 Ag suivants : CD19+, CD22+ (s ou c), cCD79a+				
	CD10	**cμ**	**s Ig**	
B-I (pro-B)	-	-	-	
B-II (common ALL)	+	-	-	
B-III (pré-B)	±	+	-	
B-IV (mature B)	±	±	+	
Pour affirmer le caractère T : cCD3+				
Ensuite on peut classer en 4 stades :	**CD7**	**CD2 et/ou CD5 et/ou CD8**	**CD1a**	**sCD3**
T-I (pro-T ou early T)	+	-	-	-
T-II (pré-T)	+	+ (au moins un)	-	-
T-III (thymocytes communs, corticaux, intermédiaires)	±	+ (au moins un) CD4+ et CD8+		±
T-IV (mature T) Groupe a : TCR % + Groupe b : TCR % +	±	+ (au moins un) CD4+ ou CD8+	-	+

Remarque : TI et TII sont parfois regroupés = thymocytes immatures ou prothymocytes.
c : cytoplasmique ; s : de surface ; Ig : immunoglobuline ; μ : chaîne lourde μ

Note: П and TH are grouped together = immature thymocytes or prothymocytes, c: cytoplasmic; s: surface; Ig: immunogtobulin; u: heavy chain p

2.3.5.2 ***Bone biopsy***

Histological analysis and immunohistochemical study are carried out if medullary aspiration is difficult. This is carried out in the anatomical pathology laboratory of the Habib Bouguiba University Hospital in Sfax.

2.3.6 ***Conventional karyotype***

Carried out on bone marrow or on blood, in the event of difficult medullary aspiration, on a lithium heparinate tube and analysed in the cytogenetics laboratory of the CHU Farhat Hached Sousse. This is used to detect any clonal chromosomal abnormalities in number and/or structure. The FISH method was not used in our series.

2.3.7 ***Searching for the bcr-abl transcript***

Performed on marrow or on blood, if medullary aspiration is difficult, on an EDTA tube and analysed in the hematology laboratory at the Institut Pasteur in Tunis using the RT-PCR method.

2.3.8 ***Study of cerebrospinal fluid***

Carried out systematically on Day 1 of prephase to look for initial neuromeningeal damage, with cytological, chemical, bacteriological and pathological examinations.

2.3.9 ***HLA typing***

Carried out at the immunology laboratory of the CHU Hedi Chaker in Sfax in search of a geno-identical HLA donor for patients with a high risk group (RE) and aged < 50 years.

2.3.10 ***Chest X-ray***

Systematically performed as part of the diagnosis to look for a mediastinal mass, pleural involvement or an infectious site.

2.4 Treatment

❖ **Non-phi+ ALLs are treated according to**:

- The Tunisian protocol, inspired by the French protocol, GRAALL 2003 between January 2005 and May 2009 (Annex N°1).
- The Tunisian protocol, inspired by the French protocol, GRAALL 2005 between June 2009 and December 2015 (Appendix 2).

The GRAALL 2003 protocol is based on a combination of polychemotherapy as follows:

J The induction treatment, common to the standard risk (STD) and high risk (RE) groups, is based on a combination of Dexamethasone, 4 injections of Oncovin, 4 injections of DNR, 6 injections of Asparaginase, 4 PL with intra-thecal injection and G-CSF from D17.

S For the STD Group :

- IB cure.
- Intermediate treatment.
- Reinduction and reconsolidation (IIA and IIB).
- Radiotherapy of the encephalon.
- Maintenance treatment.

S For the RE Group :

S Blocks B1-B2-B3, B1-B2-B3 15 days apart.

S Reinduction and reconsolidation (IIA and IIB).

S Blocks B1-B2-B3 15 days apart.

S Radiotherapy of the encephalon.

S Maintenance treatment.

S Allogeneic bone marrow transplantation for subjects aged under 40 treated according to the RE group and having a genoidentical HLA donor.

The GRAALL 2005 protocol is based on the same principles as the GRAALL 2003 protocol, with the following differences:

S Induction treatment: same schedule, with the addition of two further doses of Endoxan at a dose of 500mg/m^2 on D8 and D15.

S An extension of the indication for allogeneic bone marrow transplants to patients aged < 50 years.

❖ **Treatment of phi+ ALL** is based on a combination of chemotherapy and TKIs according to the Tunisian protocol inspired by GRAAPH 2005 (Appendix 4) (Imatinib in 1ere intention and TKI switch from 2eme generation in the event of a non-optimal response or an increase in the BCR-ABL ratio under treatment):

S Induction treatment is based on a combination of imatinib 800mg/d, dexamethasone, 3 injections of Oncovin and 3 LPs.

S Consolidation treatment is based on a combination of Imatinib 800mg/d, methotrexate (1g/m^2), high-dose aracytin (HD) and a PL with intra-thecal injection.

J A pre-transplant interphase followed by an allograft for patients aged < 50 years with a genotypic HLA donor.

J For patients without an HLA-matched donor: maintenance chemotherapy with courses combining Imatinib with Hyper CVAD-type chemotherapy, prophylactic RT of the encephalon up to C2 and maintenance treatment.

2.4.1 *Therapeutic evaluation*

2.4.1.1 *Pre-phase response*

It is assessed in non-phi+ ALL patients. It is based on determination of the absolute rate of blasts in the blood smear taken on D8 of a corticotherapie (dexamethasone) with intrathecal injection (IT) of methotrexate (MTX) on D1:

J Corticosensitivity is defined by a rate of blasts <1,000/mm^3

J Corticoresistance is defined as a rate of blasts >1,000/mm^3 (also known as poor response to corticotherapy).

2.4.1.2 *Chemosensitivity*

It is assessed for non-phi+ ALL patients. It is based on the determination of the blast rate on the medullary smear performed at D15 of induction.

Chemoresistance after 15 days of chemotherapy is defined as :

J A rate of >5% blasts on the D 15 myelogram in marrow of average or normal richness, or significant blastosis in marrow of poor or desert richness.

J And/or by a reduction of less than 75% in the peripheral tumour syndrome.

2.4.1.3 *Complete remission*

Complete remission is assessed between D30 and D35, for both non-phi+ and phi+ ALL, i.e. at the end of aplasia following induction treatment.

It is defined by :

S The disappearance of all clinical signs of the disease.

S Restoration of normal hematopoietic activity with a PNN count >1,000/mm^3 and a platelet count >100,000/mm^3

S A blast rate of less than 5% on the myelogram with a marrow of normal richness where all the lines are represented.

S Disappearance of the cytogenetic abnormalities initially found.

2.4.1.4 *Therapeutic failure:*

If one or more elements defining full remission are missing.

2.4.1.5 *Definition of risk groups :*

The stratification of our ALL cases into risk groups, according to the GRAALL 2003 and 2005 protocols, is detailed in Table II. It is based on the following criteria:

- White blood cell count at diagnosis.
- B or T immunophenotyping and degree of maturity.
- Karyotype.
- Cerebromeningeal involvement.
- Pre-phase response.
- Response after 15 days of chemotherapy.
- Obtaining CR at the end of the induction treatment.

Table II: Therapeutic stratification into risk groups according to the 2003 and 2005 Tunisian GRAALL protocols.

	GRAALL 2003	GRAALL 2005
Standard risk (STD)	No ER factors	No ER factors
High risk (ER)	- Only 1 of the following factors: - LALB - ALL with WBC>100,000/mm $.^3$ - Immature ALL (TI, TII of EGIL) - 1 (4,11) or 11q23 anomaly. - 1 (1.19), hypo diploi'die, pres triploi'die, complex karyotype (> 5 anomalies) - Neuromeningitis. - Corticoresistance at D8. - Chemoresistance at D15. - No CR after induction treatment.	- Only 1 of the following factors: - LALB with WBC>30 000/mm $.^3$ - ALL with WBC>100,000/mm $.^3$ - LAL pro B - Common LAL B. - Immature LALT. - 1 (4,11) or 11q23 anomaly. - Neuromeningitis. - Cortico-resistance at D8. - Chemoresistance at D15. - No CR after induction treatment.
LAL phi+ group	If t(9,22) and/or bcr-abl positive (result before D8).	

2.4.2 *Support treatment :*

- Hematological and biochemical monitoring tests are carried out systematically twice a week during induction treatment.
- G-CSF was administered systematically at a dose of 5 jug/kg/d from Day 17 of the induction treatment and 24 to 48 hours after the end of chemotherapy for the B1, B2 and B3 consolidation blocks.
- Depending on availability, our patients are treated in conventional isolation rooms or in rooms with 2 beds.
- All our patients benefited from alkaline hyperhydration, hypouricemic treatment during induction, antiemetic treatment and transfusions of packed red blood cells if the haemoglobin level was below 8g/dL and of platelet packed red blood cells if the platelet level was below 10,000 el/mm^3 and/or in the presence of a haemorrhagic

syndrome.

- Broad-spectrum antibiotic therapy was prescribed if the temperature was >38.2°C on a single dose or >38°C on 2 occasions. It was based on a combination of Ceftazidime or Imipenem with Amikacin. Amphotericin is reserved for cases of suspected and/or documented fungal infection, while Voriconazole is prescribed for pulmonary aspergillosis.
- Digestive decontamination with non-absorbable antibiotics is not used in our study.
- Systematic central venous catheterisation prior to each course of chemotherapy is not standard practice in our department.
- The diet of our patients is based on a protected diet.

3 Therapeutic toxicity:

It is graded according to the World Health Organisation (WHO) classification (appendix 4).

4 Study of deaths:

We studied deaths, in particular those that occurred at the time of induction and during consolidation treatment.

5 Study of relapses:

Medullary relapse is defined as the reappearance of clinical signs of disease and/or circulating blasts in the blood and/or an increase in the percentage of medullary blasts after a period of complete remission.

Neuromeningeal relapse is defined by the appearance of clinical and/or biological neuromeningeal signs.

6 Survival studies:

We have set the data cut-off date at 31 December 2017.

> **Overall survival (OS)**: is the period between the date of diagnosis and the data cut-off date, i.e. 31/12/2017, or the date of death.

> **Relapse-free survival (RFS)**: is the period from the date of CR to the date of relapse or the data cut-off date.

> **Event-free survival (EFS):** is the period between the date of diagnosis and 1er events (relapse or death) or the data cut-off date, i.e. 31/12/2017.

7 Statistical analysis:

Statistical analysis was carried out using SPSS20 software.

> **Study of correlations :**

The Chi2 (X2) test and the Kendal test were used to study correlations.

The Chi2 test is used for binary qualitative variables, and the X2 test corrects for a theoretical number of patients of less than 5.

We used Kendal's test when a variable is ordinal.

> **Survival studies :**

The Kaplan-Meier method was used to study survival.

> **Study of prognostic factors :**

The Logrank test and logistic regression were used to study prognostic factors.

3 Resutts

In the first chapter, we study the epidemiological, clinical and biological characteristics of patients treated for both phi+ and non-phi+ acute lymphoblastic leukaemia. In the second chapter, we detail the therapeutic results of the group of patients treated for non-phi+ ALL and the group of phi+ ALL patients separately.

1 Epidemiological data

1.1 Annual recruitment

We recruited 49 phi+ and non-phi+ ALL patients over 12 years, i.e. an annual recruitment of 4 cases with extremes of 1 to 8 cases/year (Figure 1).

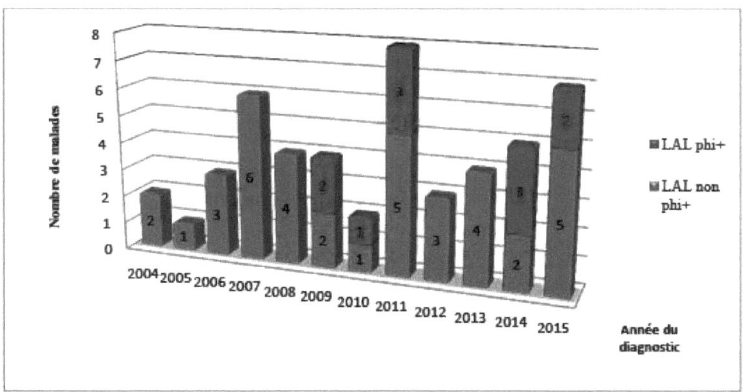

Figure 1:Number of cases of adult ALL per year.

1.2 Monthly recruitment

The distribution of our cases by month of diagnosis is shown in Figure 2. The variation in the monthly number of cases was not statistically significant (p = 0.223). The distribution of our cases was stable during the 3 seasons Spring, Winter and Summer (between 13 and 15), whereas the number of cases fell by almost half during Autumn (Figure 2).

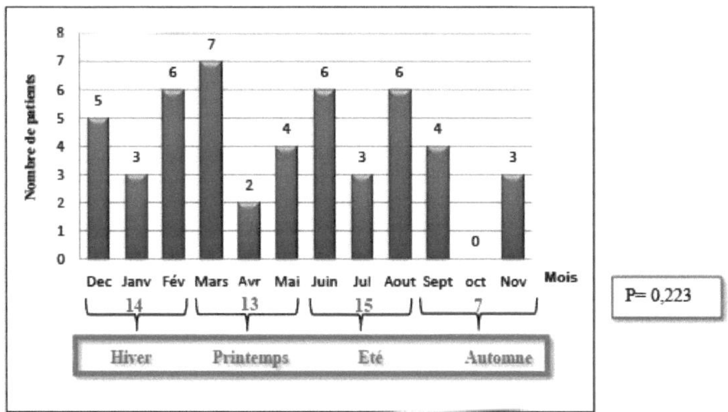

Figure 2: Number of cases of adult ALL per month.

1.3 Gender

Twenty-three patients were male (47%) and twenty-six were female (16%).
female (53%) with a sex ratio of 0.88 (Figure 3).

❖ For non-phi+ ALL patients: twenty were male (53%) and eighteen female, with a sex ratio of 1.1.

❖ For phi+ ALL patients: three male patients (27%) and eight female patients, with a sex ratio of 0.37.

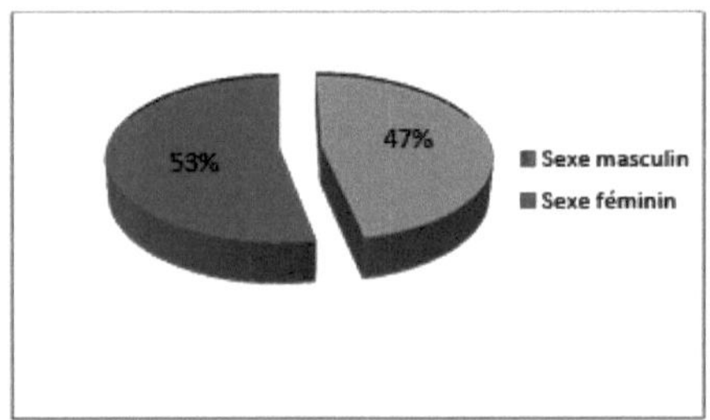

Figure 3: Gender distribution of ALL patients.

1.4 Age :

The median age at diagnosis of our patients was 42 years with extremes ranging from 20 to 56 years: the median age was 42 years (extreme 27- 56 years) for non-phi+ ALL patients and 38 years (extreme 20- 55 years) for phi+ ALL patients.

We noted a higher frequency in the 31-35 age group and in the 46-50 age group (Figure 4). Twenty-seven patients (55%) were aged over 40.

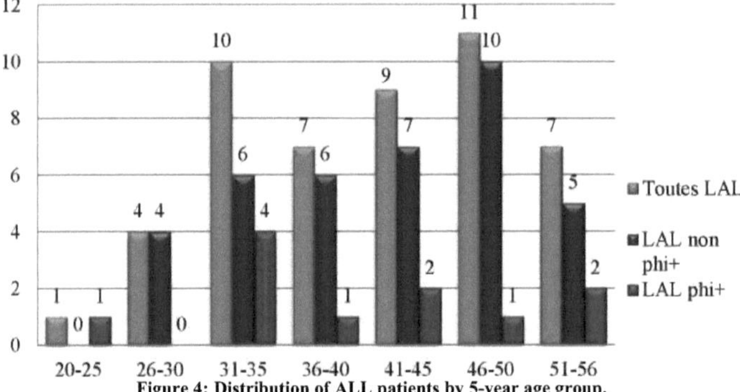

Figure 4: Distribution of ALL patients by 5-year age group.

1.5 Geographical origin:

The distribution of our patients according to geographical origin is detailed as follows (Figure 5).

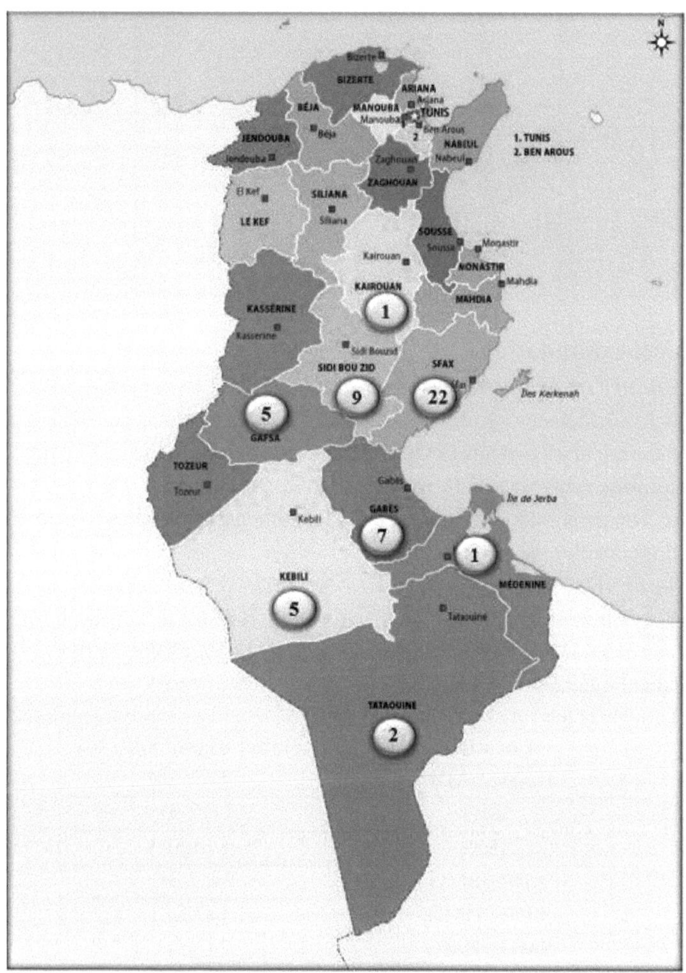

Figure 5: Breakdown of patients by geographical origin.

2 Clinical data

2.1 Reason for consultation

Anaemic syndrome was the most frequent reason for consultation in 29 patients (59%), followed by infectious syndrome (11 patients, 22%) and haemorrhagic syndrome (11 patients, 22%). Tumour syndrome was the reason for consultation in seven patients (19.5%).

2.2 Consultation deadline :

The average consultation time was 30 days, with extremes ranging from 3 to 90 days (Figure 6).

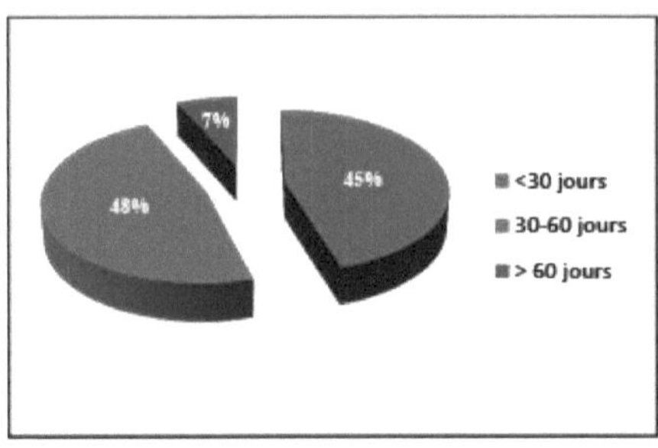

Consultation period in days.

2.3 Clinical examination

2.3.1 *Medullary insufficiency syndrome*

A medullary insufficiency syndrome was present in 43 patients, i.e. 88% of cases: an anemic syndrome in 41 patients (84%), a haemorrhagic syndrome in 13 patients (26%) and an infectious syndrome in 16 patients (32%). An infectious site was identified in 11 patients. The most frequent sites were ENT, pulmonary and cutaneous in 36%, 27% and 18% respectively.

2.3.2 *Tumour syndrome*

A tumour syndrome was noted in 31 patients (63%). It consisted of isolated adenopathies in 35.5% and isolated splenomegaly in 22.5% (Table N°III).

Mediastinal enlargement was found in 8 cases, i.e. 16% of cases.

Table III: Location of tumour syndrome in our patients.

Location	Number of patients (%)
Isolated ADP	11 (35,5)
SMG	7 (22,5)
HMG	1 (3,5)
ADP+ SMG	7 (22,5)
ADP+ HMG	1 (3,5)
SMG+ HMG	2 (6,5)
ADP+ SMG+ HMG	2 (6,5)
Total	31 (100%)

2.3.3 *Damage to the central nervous system:*

Initial involvement of the central nervous system was noted in 3 patients (5%), clinical in 2 and biological in all.

In the case of the patient whose CSF showed no blasts, a cerebral MRI scan was carried out, revealing pachymeningitis.

The clinico-biological characteristics of these 3 patients are detailed in table N°IV:

Table IV: Clinical and biological characteristics of patients with initial neuromeningeal disease.

Age (Years)	Gender	IPT	GB /mm3	Karyotype	Clinic	CSF
32	M	T	3800	Normal	Paralysis of the right VI,	Hyper proteinorrachia

				(Nle)	cerebellar syndrome, hypoesthesia of the hoop	No blasts
53	M	B	7800	Nle	Normal	Presence of blasts
29	M	T	4900	Non Informative (NI)	Left VI paralysis hypoesthesia of the hoop	Presence of blasts

2.3.4 ***Testicular damage :***

No patient was diagnosed with testicular involvement.

3 Biological characteristics :

3.1 Blood count :

3.1.1 ***Initial leukocytosis:***

The median white blood cell count in our patients was 10,000/mm^3 (extreme 560/mm^3 -385 600/mm).^{3}

Leukocytosis of less than 30,000/mm^3 was noted in 35 patients (72%), eight patients (16%) had leukocytosis between 30,000 and 100,000 and hyperleukocytosis >100,000/mm^3 was noted in 6 cases (12%) (Figure 7).

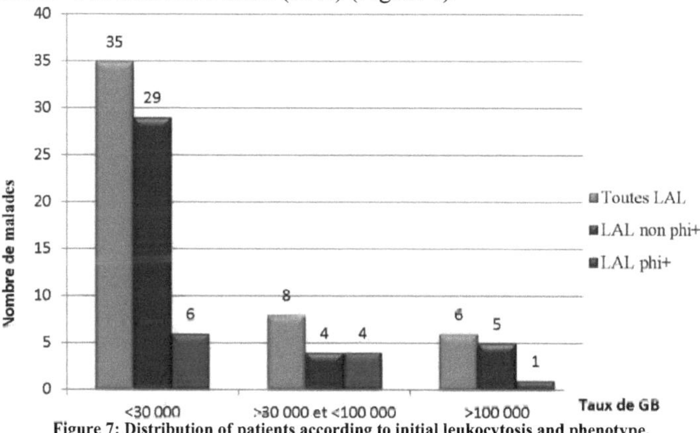

Figure 7: Distribution of patients according to initial leukocytosis and phenotype.

3.1.2 ***Blood blastosis:***

Blood blastosis was observed in 38 patients (77%), with the percentage of blasts in the blood ranging from 2% to 99% (median 25%).

3.1.3 ***Haemoglobin levels:***

The median hemoglobin level was 7.5 g/dL with extremes from 2.4 g/dL to 14.6 g/dL. A hemoglobin level < 10 g/dL was found in 36 patients (73%).

3.1.4 ***Number of wafers:***

The median platelet count was 40,000/mm3 (ranging from 3,000/mm^3 to 341,000/mm^3). Thrombocytopenia was observed in 43 patients, or 87% of cases. Thrombocytopenia was less than 50,000 in 59% of cases.

3.2 Hemostasis check-up:

Biological DIC was observed in only one patient (2%).

3.3 Tumour lysis syndrome

Spontaneous tumour lysis syndrome occurred in five patients (10%), three of whom had WBC levels >100 G/L.

3.4 Myelogram:

It was carried out in all patients, showing blastic infiltration > 20% in all cases.

3.5 Immunophenotyping:

LPT by flow cytometry was performed in 44 patients (90% of cases) and by BOM with immunohistochemical study in 5 patients (10% of cases).

At the end of this study, B-phenotype ALL was found in 32 cases (65%), T-phenotype ALL in 16 cases (33%) and biphenotypic acute leukaemia (B + myeloid) in one case (2%) (Table V).

All phi+ ALL were of B phenotype (including 8 common B ALL, one pre-B ALL and one biphenotypic ALL).

Table V: Phenotype distribution of our ALL patients.

	LAL B (%)	LAL T (%)	Biphenotypic LA (%)	Total
Non-phi+ ALL	22 (58)	16 (42)	0	38
LAL phi+	10 (90)	0	1 (10)	11
Total	32 (65)	16 (33)	1(2)	49

3.6 Cytogenetic study:

The cytogenetic study carried out on 47 patients, i.e. 90% of cases, was conclusive in only 33 patients.

Of these 33 karyotypes, 16 (49%) were normal whereas cytogenetic abnormalities were found in 17 cases (51%). T (9,22) was found in 6 cases (Figure 8).

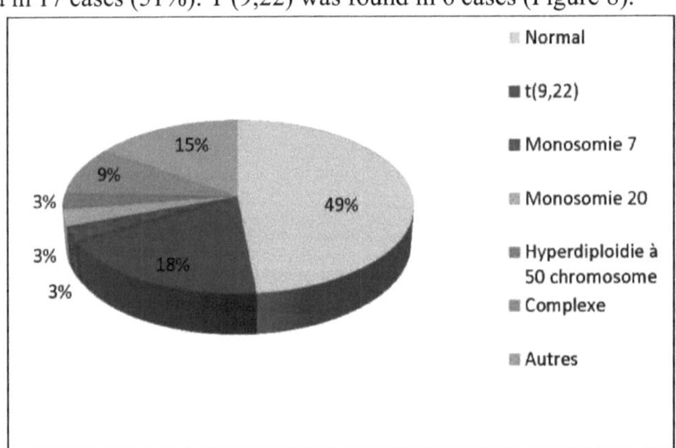

Figure 8: Distribution of cytogenetic abnormalities in patients.

3.7 Molecular biology:

Bcr-Abl transcript testing was performed in 45 patients. It was positive in 10 cases (22%). One patient had t (9.22) with a negative Bcr-Abl transcript.

The transcript type was e1a2 in 7 cases, b3a2 in 2 cases and b2a2 in 1 case: i.e. p190 in 7 cases and p210 in 3 cases.

4 Therapeutic results :

4.1 Distribution of our patients according to chemotherapy protocols:

Of the 49 patients, only 46 received adequate treatment:

> One patient was not treated because of associated comorbidities (suspected thyroid nodule, extensive left popliteal thrombophlebitis).

> Two patients were treated outside the protocol: one patient received prephase and was then lost to follow-up for 4 months, while the second patient received a CHOP treatment before prephase (treated in the city for B lymphoma, but the diagnosis was later rectified).

The 46 patients treated were:

> Non-phi+ ALL treated according to the protocol in 36 patients.

> LAL treated according to the LAL phi+ protocol in 10 patients.

The chemotherapy protocol used is detailed in Table VI.

Table VI: Chemotherapy protocol used for our patients.

Chemotherapy protocol	January 2004- May 2009	June 2009- December 2015	
	GRAALL 2003	GRAALL 2005	GRAAPH 2005
Number of patients	17	19	10

4.2 Therapeutic results of patients followed for non-phi+ ALL:

4.2.1 *Pre-phase response:*

A smear was taken on day 8 for all patients: 32 patients were corticosensitive (89%) and 4 patients were corticoresistant (11%).

The study of the factors influencing the response to the prephase showed :

In univariate analysis, only the WBC count (<10,000) had a significant influence on prephase response ($p=0.04$). The absence of a tumour syndrome, B phenotype and age appeared to influence response to prephase but not significantly (p= 0.141; 0.125 and 0.287 respectively).

In multivariate analysis, no factor significantly influenced corticosensitivity (Table VII).

Table VII: Factors influencing prephase response.

		FS<1000/mm^3 (%)	P Uni variee	P Multi variee
Age	<40 years (n=15) >40 years (n=21)	12 (80) 20 (95)	0,287	0,547
Gender	Male (n=19) Female (n=17)	17 (89,5) 15 (88)	1	0 ,998
Tumour syndrome	Yes (n=22) No (n=14)	18 (88) 14 (100)	0,141	0,999
GB	<30000/mm^3 (n=27) >30000/mm^3 (n=9)	24 (75) 8 (75)	0,99	-

	<10000/mm^3 (n=19) >10000/mm^3 (n=1?)	19(100) 13 (76,5)	**0,04**	0,997
	<30000/mm^3 (n=27) >30000 and <100000/mm^3 (n=4) >1000000/mm^3 (n=5)	24 (89) 4 (100) 4 (80)	0,902	-
Phenotype	B (n=21) T (n=15)	17 (81) 15 (100)	0,125	0,997
Karyotype	Normal (n=14) Abnormal (n=10)	13 (93) 11 (70)	0,272	-

4.2.2 *Chemosensitivity:*

Sternal puncture at D15 was performed in 29 patients: 24 were chemosensitive (83%) and 5 chemoresistant (17%).

The study of factors influencing chemosensitivity showed that corticosensitivity had a significant influence on chemosensitivity at D15 in univariate analysis with a significant p-value at 0.01 (Table VIII).

In multivariate analysis, no factor significantly influenced chemosensitivity at day 15.

Table VIII: Factors influencing response to chemosensitivity.

		Chemosensitivity (%)	**P Univarie**	**P Multivarie**
Age	<40 years (n=14) >40 years (n=15)	11(79) 13 (87)	0,651	0,665
Gender	Male (n=17) Female (n=12)	14 (82) 10 (83)	1	0,806
Tumour Syndrome	Yes (n=20) No (n=9)	16 (80) 8 (89)	1	0,999
GB	<30000/mm^3 (n=19) >30000/mm^3 (n=10)	15(79) 9 (90)	0,633	-
	<10000/mm^3 (n=13) >10000/mm^3 (n=16)	11 (85) 13(81)	1	0,999
	<30000/mm^3 (n=20) >30000 and <100000/mm^3 (n=4) >100000/mm^3 (n=5)	16 (80) 4 (100) 4 (80)	0,662	-
Corticosensitivity	Yes (n=25) No (n=4)	23 (92) 1 (25)	**0,01**	0,998
Phenotype	B (n=15) T(n=14)	12 (80) 12 (86)	1	-
Karyotype	Normal (n=12) Abnormal (n=9)	10 (83) 6 (67)	0,611	-

4.2.3 *Study of complete remission:*

4.2.3.1 *Overall assessment :*

Four patients (11%) died during the induction treatment and before re-evaluation.

Of the 32 evaluable patients, 29 were in CR after an induction treatment, i.e. 90% of cases, and 1 patient was in CR after 2 courses of chemotherapy, i.e. an overall CR rate of 93% (30 patients). If we included patients who had undergone induction in the

evaluation of remission, the overall CR rate would be 83%.
Two patients (5%) had failed treatment after two courses of chemotherapy.
The clinico-biological characteristics of patients who have failed a treatment are detailed in table IX.

Table IX: Characteristics of patients who failed after induction (one course).

Age (years)	Gender	Tumour Sd	GB G/L	Hb g/dL	Plq G/L	Phenotype	Karyotype	FS J8	PS J15	2nd Induction	2nd RC
53	M	No	7,8	5,5	24	B	Nle	<1000	<5%	Arac+ Novantrone	Yes
29	M	No	4,9	9	13	T	NI	<1000	<5%	Arac+ Novantrone	No
50	M	No	9,3	7,1	54	B	Nle	<1000	Hemo-diluted	Arac+ DNR	No

4.2.3.2 *Study of the various factors influencing the achievement of CR:*

No factor significantly influenced CR. Sex, absence of tumour syndrome and chemotherapy protocol appeared to influence complete remission without the difference being significant (p=0.492; 0.131 and 0.212 respectively) (Table X).

Table X: Factors influencing CR.

		RC (%)	P in univarie
Age	<40 years (n=15) >40 years (n=17)	14 (93) 16 (94)	1
Gender	Male (n=18) Female (n=14)	16 (89) 14 (100)	0,492
Tumour syndrome	Yes (n=20) No (n=12)	20(100) 10 (83)	0,131
GB	<30000/mm^3 (n=24) >30000/mm^3 (n=8)	22 (92) 8(100)	1
	<10000/mm^3 (n=18) >10000/mm^3 (n=14)	16 (89) 14 (100)	0,492
	<30000/mm^3 (n=25) >30000 and <100000/mm^3 (n=3) >100000/mm^3 (n=4)	23 (92) 3(100) 4(100)	0,173
Phenotype	B (n=18) T (n=14)	16 (94,5) 13 (93)	1
Karyotype	Normal (n=13) Abnormal (n=9)	12 (92) 9(100)	1
Corticosensitivity	<1000/mm3 (n=28) >1000/mm3 (n=4)	26(93) 4(100)	1
Chemosensitivity	Yes (n=22) No (n=5)	21 (95,5) 5(100)	1
Asparaginase injection (ASPA)	<2 injections (n=10) >2 injections (n=18)	10 (100) 16 (89)	0,524
	<3 injections (n=19) >3 injections (n=9)	18(95) 8 (89)	1

Chemotherapy protocol	GRAALL 2003 (n=15) GRAALL 2005 (n=16)	13 (87) 16 (100)	0,212

4.2.4 *Therapeutic stratification according to risk group*

The stratification of ALL patients into risk groups is as follows: > Standard risk group = 7 cases (20%).

> High risk group = 29 cases (80%).

The stratification of the 30 CR patients is as follows:

> Standard risk group = 6 cases.

> High risk group = 24 cases including :

- B-phenotype ALL = 15 cases
- T-phenotype ALL = 9 cases

S LAL T with WBC > 100 000/mm^3 = 3 cases.

S T-ALL with immature phenotype = 4 cases.

Chemoresistant T-ALL = 1 case.

T-ALL with neuromeningeal involvement = 1 case.

4.2.5 *Study of deaths:*

We have recorded 23 deaths in our series.

4.2.5.1 *Induction defects :*

Seven patients (19%) died during induction treatment:

S Four have died before therapeutic evaluation.

S A patient died in complete remission.

S Two patients failed after 2 courses of chemotherapy due to disease progression.

The time between death and the start of treatment ranged from 15 to 37 days, with a median of 26 days (Table XI).

Table XI: Characteristics of induction patients.

Age (years)	Gender	Tumour sd	GB G/L	IPT	Gpe Ttt	Karyotype	Chemosensitivity	Hematological status	Deadline	Cause of death
45	F	No	230	T	RE	Nle	Yes	NE	J 26	Septic shock
51	M	Yes	10	B	RE	NI	HD	NE	J 24	Multivisor failure
47	M	No	0,9	B	RE	NI	HD	NE	J 15	Septic shock
50	F	Yes	56	B	RE	Complex	Yes	NE	J 33	OAP lesionnel
40	F	Yes	98	B	RE	Complex	Yes	RC	J 37	Hemorrhagic shock
29	M	No	4,9	T	STD	NI	Yes	Failure	-	Evolution of the disease
50	M	No	9,3	B	RE	Nle	HD	Failure	-	Evolution of the disease

*Death due to profuse hemoptysis secondary to angioinvasive pulmonary aspergillosis.

**Hemodiluee (HD).

4.2.5.2 *Dices in consolidation :*

Three patients (10%) died during consolidation treatment:

J Two post-bone marrow allograft patients with GVH in 1 case and hepatitis B reactivation in one case.

J One patient died during maintenance treatment for septic shock (Table XII).

Table XII: Characteristics of patients who died during consolidation.

Age (years)	Gender	Tumour sd	GB G/L	IPT	Gpe tt	Karyotype	Chemosensitivity	Induction response	Phase ttt	Cause of death
47	F	No	1,2	T	RE	T 4	HD	RC	Post-transplant	GVH
45	M	No	6,5	T	RE	Nle	No	RC	5 years post-transplant	Reactivation hepatitis B
30	F	No	2,4	B	RS	Nle	Yes	RC	Maintenance	Septic shock

4.2.5.3 *Dices par ivolutiviti de la maladie*

During follow-up, thirteen deaths were recorded in our series due to progression of the disease.

4.2.6 *Study of relapses*

Of the 30 patients in CR, 2 did not complete their treatments: one patient died after induction due to hemorrhagic shock and one patient was lost to follow-up after induction.

4.2.6.1 *Frequency and duration of relapses*

Fourteen patients relapsed during the study period out of the 28 CR patients who continued their treatment, i.e. 50% of cases:

S Three cases (50%) were treated according to the standard risk group

S Eleven cases (50%) in the high-risk group (Table XIII).

The average time to relapse was 9 months (2 - 31 months).

Seventy-one per cent of relapses occurred within 1ere year of CR, i.e. during the course of treatment. The latest relapse occurred 31 months after CR.

Table XIII: Frequency and mean time to relapse according to risk group.

	Total number (%)	RC (%)	Relapse (%)	Average time (months)
Standard risk	7 (20)	6 (22)	3 (50)	20
High risk	29 (80)	22 (78)	11 (50)	6
Total	36 (100)	28 (100)	14 (100)	9

4.2.6.2 *Location and characteristics of relapsed patients*

Isolated medullary relapse was the most common site, occurring in 79% of cases, followed by combined medullary and neuromeningeal relapse in 14% of cases.

Isolated neuromeningeal relapse was observed in only one case.

No patient had a testicular relapse (Table XIV).

Table XIV: Different types of relapse and their frequency.

	Number of patients (%)
Isolated medullary	11 (79)
Isolated neuromeningitis	1 (7)
Combined (Medullary + neuro-meningeal)	2 (14)

Total	14 (100)

The clinico-biological characteristics of patients who relapsed are detailed in table XV.

Table XV: Characteristics of patients who relapsed.

Age (years)	Gender	GB G/L	IPT	Gpe ttt	Karyotype	Cortico sensitivity	Chemosensitivity	Protocol	Induction response	RC/ Relapse	Relapse site	State NMS
53	M	7,8	B	RE	Nle	Yes	Yes	GRAALL 2003	RC	1 month	Meningee	DCD
31	F	140	B	RE	Nle	No	No	GRAALL 2003	RC	3 months	Medullary	DCD
29	M	4,1	T	RE	HyperD 50 hp	Yes	No	GRAALL 2003	RC	6 months	Medullary	DCD
32	M	3,8	T	RE	Nle	Yes	Yes	GRAALL 2003	RC	8 months	Medullary Meningee	DCD
27	M	10,3	B	RE	error 13 and 14	No	No	GRAALL 2003	RC	13 months	Medullary	DCD
50	M	1,5	T	RS	complex	Yes	Yes	GRAALL 2003	RC	14 months	Medullary	DCD
43	M	59	T	RS	t (15,18) der15	Yes	Yes	GRAALL 2003	RC	16 months	Medullary	DCD
32	M	4,5	T	RS	NI	Yes	Yes	GRAALL 2003	RC	31 months	Medullary	DCD
39	F	3,77	B	RE	Nle	Yes	NI	GRAALL 2005	RC	2 months	Medullary	VV
53	M	119	T	RE	NI	Yes	Yes	GRAALL 2005	RC	3 months	Medullary Meningee	DCD
50	F	4,4	B	RE	NI	Not done	NI	GRAALL 2005	RC	3 months	Medullary	DCD
45	F	16,4	B	RE	Nle	Yes	Yes	GRAALL 2005	RC	3 months	Medullary	DCD
42	F	214	B	RE	T(12,14)	No	No	GRAALL 2005	RC	5 months	Medullary	DCD
32	M	335	T	RE	Nle	Yes	Yes	GRAALL 2005	RC	12 months	Medullary	DCD

4.2.6.3 *Factors influencing the occurrence of relapse :*

Allogeneic bone marrow transplantation was the only statistically significant factor influencing the absence of relapse in our series. Corticoresistance at D8, chemoresistance at D15 and the GRAALL 2003 protocol appear to influence the occurrence of relapse, with relapse rates of 75 vs 46%, 80 vs 40% and 61.5 vs 40% respectively, without the difference being statistically significant.

This could be explained by the small size of our series (Table XVI).

Table XVI: Factors influencing the occurrence of relapses.

		Relapse (%)	P univarie
Age	<40 years (n=13) >40 years (n=15)	7 (54) 7 (47)	0,705
Gender	Male (n=16) Female (n=12)	9 (56) 5 (42)	0,445
Tumour syndrome	Yes (n=19) No (n=9)	11 (58) 3 (33)	0,420
GB	<30 000 (n=21)	10(48) 4 (57)	1

	>30 000 (n=7)		
	<10 000 (n=15) >10 000 (n=13)	7 (47) 7 (54)	0,705
Phenotype	B (n=15) T (n=13)	7 (47) 7 (54)	0,705
Karyotype	Normal (n=12) Abnormal (n=10)	7 (58) 7 (62)	1
Corticosensitivity	<1000/mm3 (n=24) >1000/mm3 (n=4)	11(46) 3 (75)	0,596
Chemosensitivity	Yes (n=20) No (n=5)	8(40) 4 (80)	0,160
Risk group	Standard risk (n=6) High risk (n=22)	3 (50) 11(50)	1
Injection of ASPA	<2 injections (n=10) >2 injections (n=15)	7 (70) 6 (40)	0,226
	<3 injections (n=17) >3 injections (n=8)	9 (53) 4 (50)	1
Chemotherapy protocol	GRAALL 2003 (n=13) GRAALL 2005 (n=15)	8 (61,5) 6 (40)	0,256
Allograft	Yes (n=9) No (n=17)	1 (11) 11 (65)	**0,014**

4.2.6.4 *Treatment of relapses*

Of the fourteen patients who relapsed, only three received catch-up treatment (Figure 9):

S Two patients received catch-up treatment with high-dose aracytin combined with novantrone, resulting in a 2eme CR, and both underwent allogeneic transplantation. One patient was alive with CR until the date of last news and the second died post allograft from GVH.

S A patient presented with a combined medullary and neuro meningeal relapse treated with radiotherapy of the encephalon in association with chemotherapy, with rapid death due to progression of the disease.

The remaining eleven patients were not treated due to poor general condition at relapse and/or lack of an HLA-matched donor and/or early relapse and all died of progressive disease.

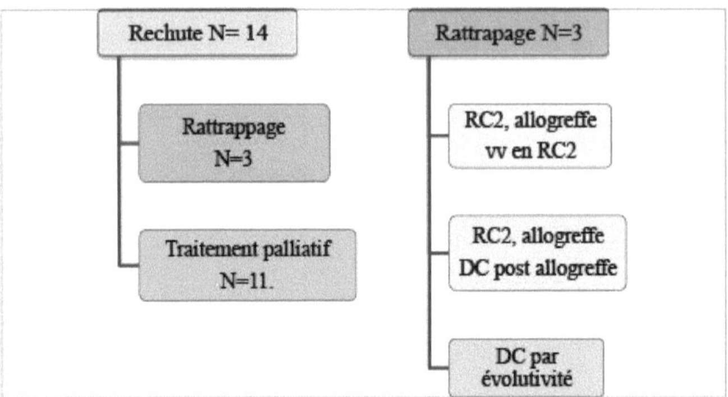

Figure 9: Trend in patients who relapsed.

4.2.7 *Bone marrow allograft :*

Among the 28 patients in CR who continued their treatment :

- Twenty patients were indicated for allogeneic transplantation (the remaining 8 = 2 patients aged > 50 years and 6 at risk of STD).
- Fourteen had an HLA-matched donor (70%).
- Nine were allografted in RC1 with a median delay of 15 weeks:
- The transplant was not carried out in 5 patients because of :

S Age 50 +/- comorbidities = 2 cases.

S Relapse before allograft = 2 cases.

S Comorbidities =1 case.

- Two patients were allografted in RC2 (STD =1 and RE =1). (Figure 10).

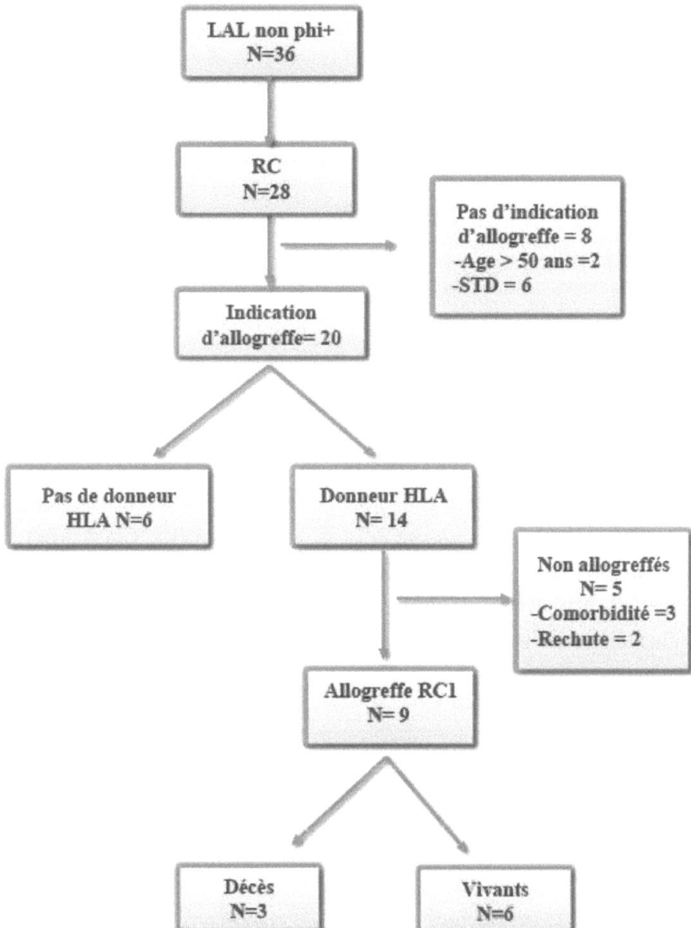

Figure 10: Feasibility of allogeneic bone marrow transplantation in non-phi+ ALL.

4.2.8 *Survival study*

The average follow-up in our series was 92 months (24 to 159 months).

4.2.8.1 *Overall survival*

The overall survival rate for the entire population was 60% at 1 year, 43% at 2 years and 36% at 5 years (Figure 11).

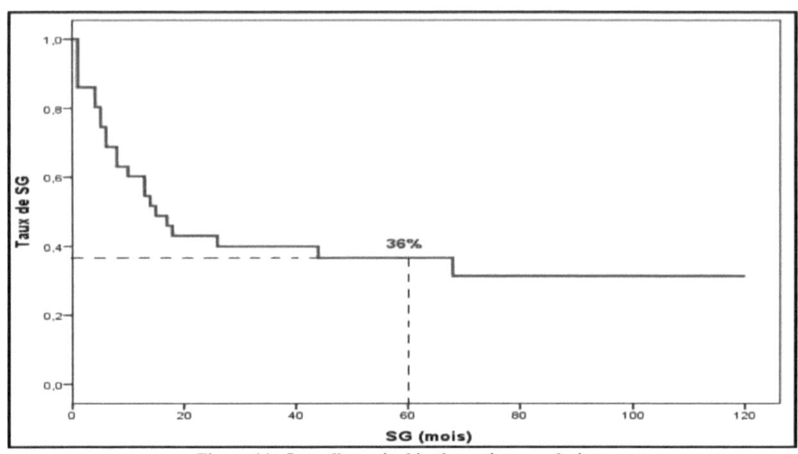

Figure 11: Overall survival in the entire population.

> ***Study of factors influencing overall survival :***

Allogeneic bone marrow transplantation was the only significant factor influencing OS in our series in both univariate and multivariate analysis with a significant p of 0.007 and 0.018 respectively. Chemosensitivity, chemotherapy protocol and age appear to be factors influencing OS but not significantly (0.133, 0.230 and 0.312 respectively) (Table XVII):

Table XVII: Factors influencing SG.

		SG is 5 years old	P univariee	P multivariee
Age	< 40 years (n=15) > 40 years (n=21)	40 35	0, 312	0,787
Gender	Male (n=19) F6min (n=17)	36 37	0,762	0,790
Tumour syndrome	Yes (n=22) No (n=14)	35 39	0,864	-
GB	<30000/mm^3 (n=26) >30000 /mm^3 (n=10)	41 25	0,492	-
	<10000/mm^3 (n=19) >10000 /mm^3 (n=17)	37 35	0,700	-
IPT	B (n=21) T (n=15)	39 32	0,925	-
Karyotype	Normal (n=14) Abnormal (n=10)	35 21	0,549	-
Blastosis j8	<1000/mm^3 (n=32) >1000/mm^3 (n=4)	38 25	0,696	-
Chemosensitivity	Yes (n=24) No (n=5)	44 20	0,133	0,053
Treatment protocol	GRAALL 2003 (n=17)	23	0,230	-

	GRAALL 2005 (n=19)	50		
ASPA injection	<2 injections (n=14) >=2 injections (n=18)	26 47	0,410	-
	<3 injections (n=23) >=3 injections (n=9)	36 44	0,600	-
Risk group	Standard risk (n=7) High risk (n=29)	28 40	0,613	-
Allograft	Yes (n=9) No (n=25)	77 21	0,013	0,018

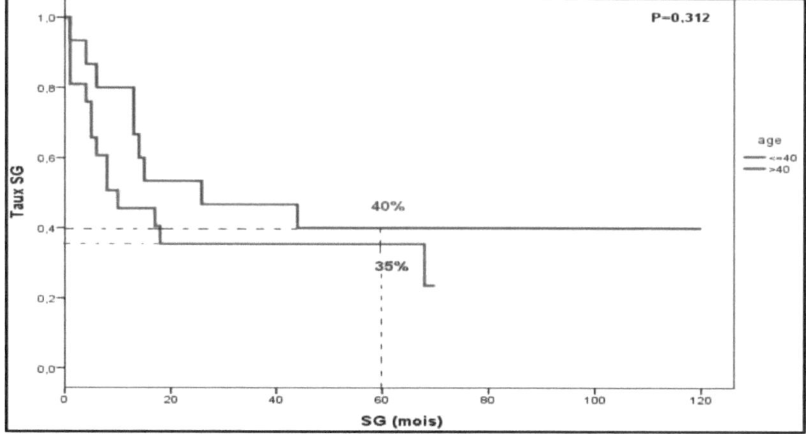

Figure 12: Overall survival as a function of Page.

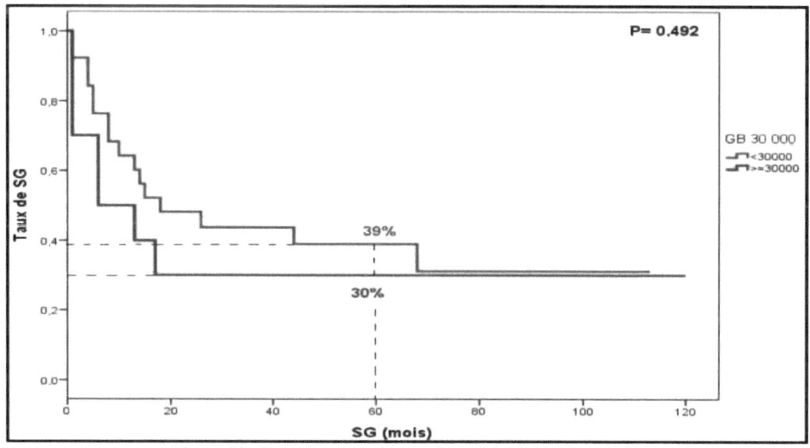

Figure 13: Overall survival according to initial leukocytosis.

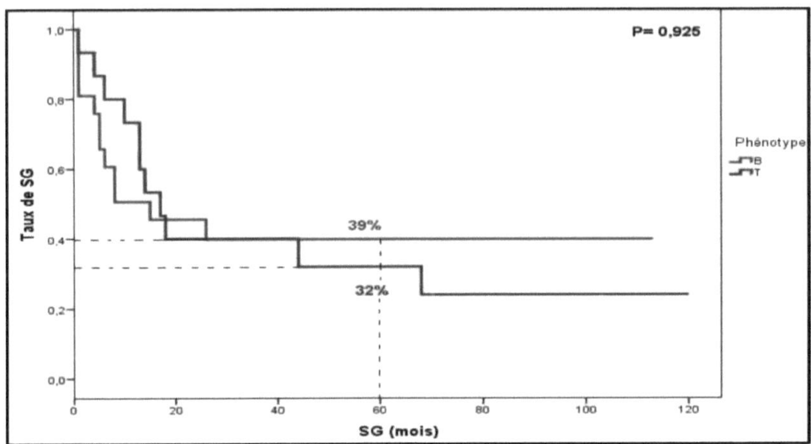

Figure 14: Overall survival as a function of phenotype.

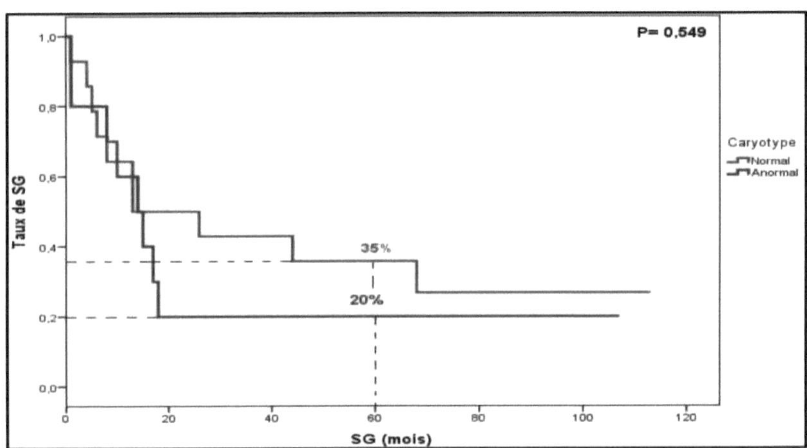

Figure 15: Overall survival according to initial karyotype.

Figure 16: Overall survival as a function of corticosteroid sensitivity.

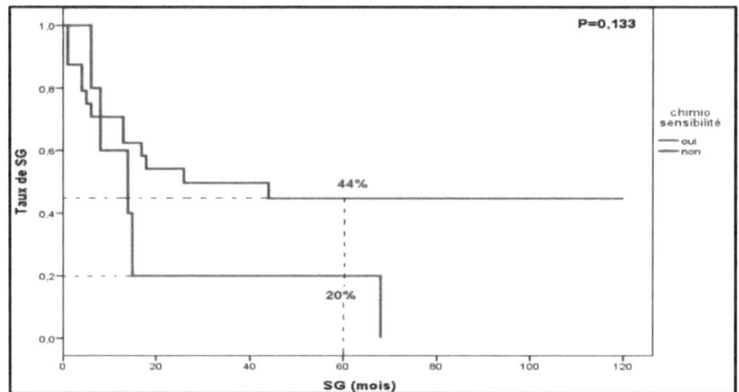

Figure 17: Overall survival according to chemosensitivity at D15.

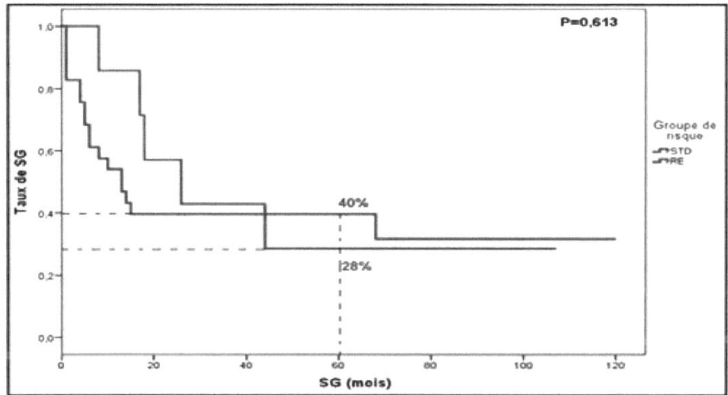

Figure 18: Overall survival according to risk group.

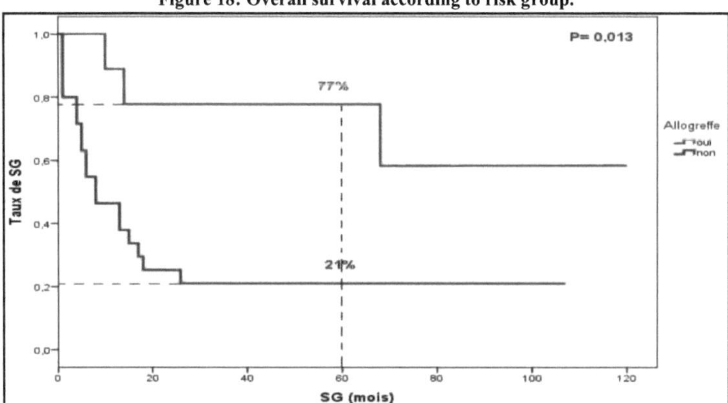

Figure 19: Overall survival according to allograft.

4.2.8.2 *Relapse-free survival :*

The SRH was 67% at 1 year. It was only 52% and 47% at 2 and 5 years respectively (Figure 20).

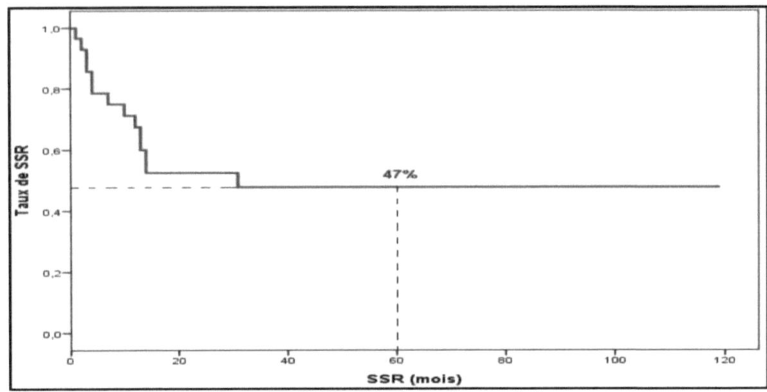

Figure 20: SRH within the entire population.

> ***Study of the factors influencing SRH :***

In univariate analysis, chemosensitivity, absence of tumour syndrome and allogeneic transplantation were the only statistically significant factors influencing SRH in our series, with p values of 0.05, 0.028 and 0.019 respectively. Corticosensitivity and initial leukocytosis appeared to influence SRH but not significantly (0.224 and 0.223 respectively).

In multivariate analysis, chemosensitivity and allografting had a statistically significant influence on SSR, with p values of 0.041 and 0.020 respectively (Table XVIII).

Table XVIII: Factors influencing SRH.

		SSR at 5 years old % of SSR at 5 years old % of SSR at 5 years old	**P univariee**	**P multivariee**
Age	<40 years (n= 13) >40 years (n= 15)	45 52	0,906	0,474
Gender	Male (n= 16) Fëminin (n= 12)	42 58	0,897	0,687
Tumour syndrome	Yes (n= 6) No (n= 19)	0 62	**0,028**	0,397
GB	<10000/mm^3 (n= 15) >100000/mm^3 (n= 13)	48 46	0,851	-
	<30000/mm^3 (n= 21) >30000/mm^3 (n= 7)	49 42	0,812	-
	<100,000/mm^3 (n= 24) >100,000/mm^3 (n= 4)	51 25	0,223	-
Phenotype	B (n= 15) T(n= 13)	53 40	0,954	-
Karyotype	Normal (n= 12) Abnormal (n= 8)	40 29	0,978	-
FS j8	<1000/mm^3 (n= 24)	51	0,244	-

	>1000/mm^3 (n= 4)	25		
Chemosensitivity at D15	Yes (n= 20) No (n= 5)	58 20	**0,05**	**0,022**
Chemotherapy protocol	GRAALL 2003 (n= 13) GRAALL 2005 (n= 15)	37 60	0,507	-
ASPA injection	<2 injections (n= 10) >=2 injections (n= 12)	26 59	0,613	-
	<3 injections (n= 17) >=3 injections (n= 8)	44 50	0,918	-
Risk group	Standard risk (n= 6) High risk (n= 22)	44 49	0,554	-
Allograft	Yes (n= 9) No (n= 17)	87 35	**0,019**	**0,041**

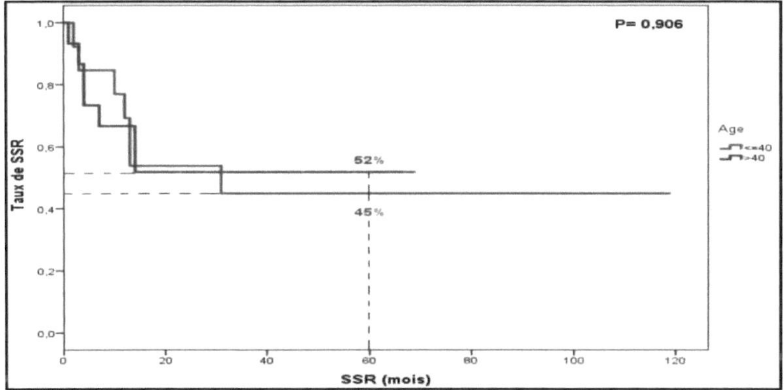

Figure 21: SSR by age.

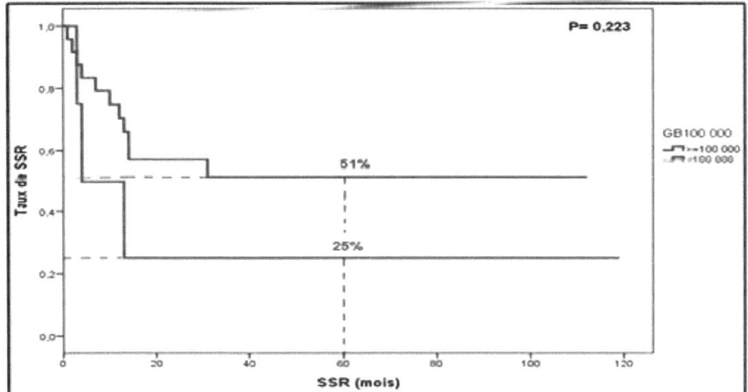

Figure 22: SSR as a function of GB.

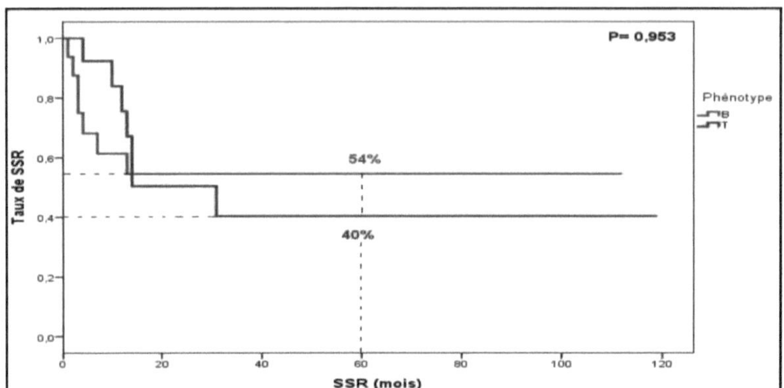

Figure 23: SSR as a function of phenotype.

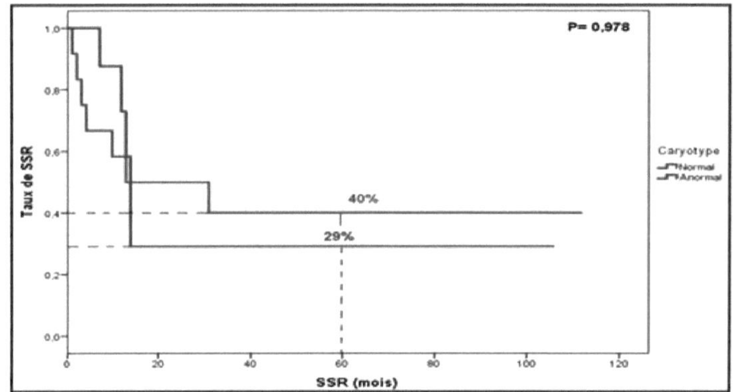

Figure 24: SSR according to initial karyotype.

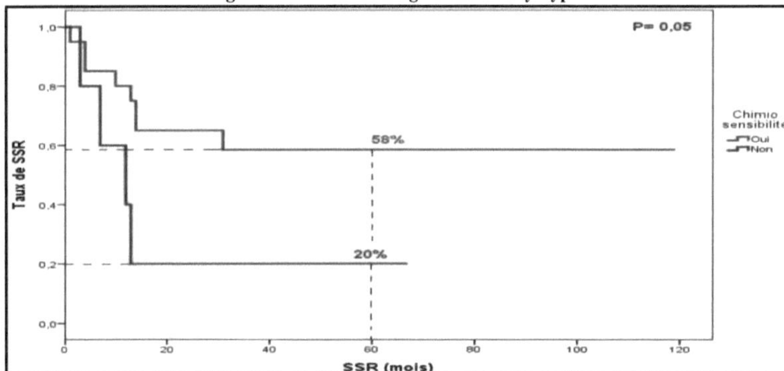

Figure 25: SSR as a function of chemosensitivity.

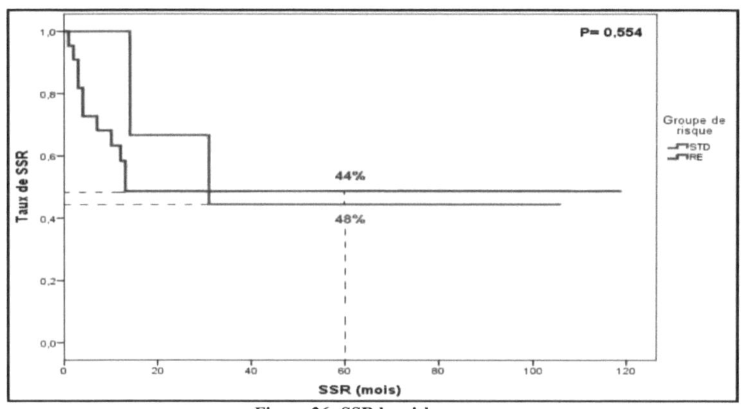

Figure 26: SSR by risk group.

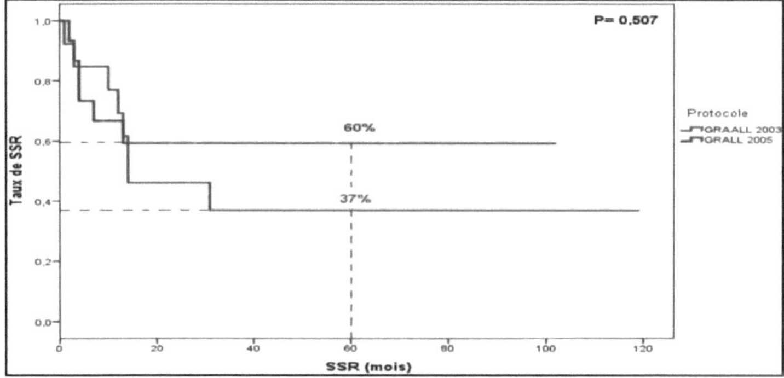

Figure 27: SSR according to therapeutic protocol.

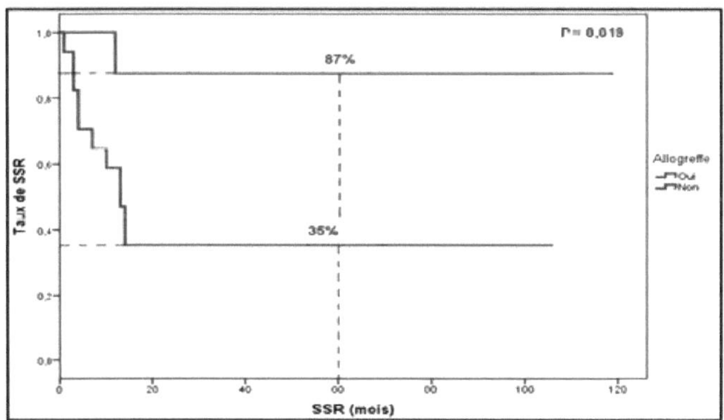

Figure 28: SSR according to allograft.

4.2.8.3 *Event-free survival:*

The SES was 50% at 1 year. It was only 38% and 35% at 2 and 5 years respectively (Figure 29).

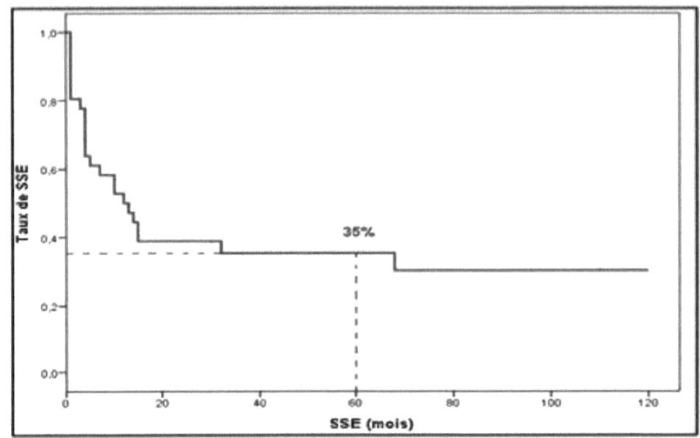

Figure 29: SES within the entire population.

> ***Study of the factors influencing SES :***

In univariate and multivariate analysis, allogeneic bone marrow transplantation was the only significant factor influencing SES in our series (p= 0.017 and 0.036 respectively). Chemosensitivity, the number of asparaginase injections and age appear to be factors influencing SES but not significantly (0.109 and 0.311 and 0.310 respectively) (table XIX).

Table XIX: Factors influencing SES.

		SSE is 5 years old	P Univariee	P Multivariee
Age	<40 years (n=15) >40 years (n=21)	39 33	0,310	0,520
Gender	Male (n=19) Female (n=17)	36 35	0,510	0,908
Tumour syndrome	Yes (n=22) No (n=14)	35 35	0,503	-
GB	<30000/mm³ (n=27) 30000 to 100000/mm³ (n=4) >100000/mm³ (n=5)	39 25 20	0,636	-
Phenotype	B (n=21) T (n=15)	38 32	0,827	-
Karyotype	Normal (n=14) Abnormal (n=10)	34 20	0,757	-
Corticosensbilite	<1000/mm³ (n=32) >1000/mm³ (n=4)	36 25	0,872	-
Chemosensitivity at D15	Yes (n=24) No (n=5)	48 20	0,109	0,068
Chemotherapy protocol	GRAALL 2003 (n=17) GRAALL 2005 (n=19)	28 42	0,636	-
Injection ASPA	<2 injections (n=14) >=2 injections (n=18)	19 44	0,311	-
	<3 injections (n=23) >=3 injections (n=9)	30 44	0,421	-

Risk group	Standard (n=7) High risk (n=29)	38 34	0,337	-
Allograft	Yes (n=9) No (n=25)	77 24	**0,017**	**0,036**

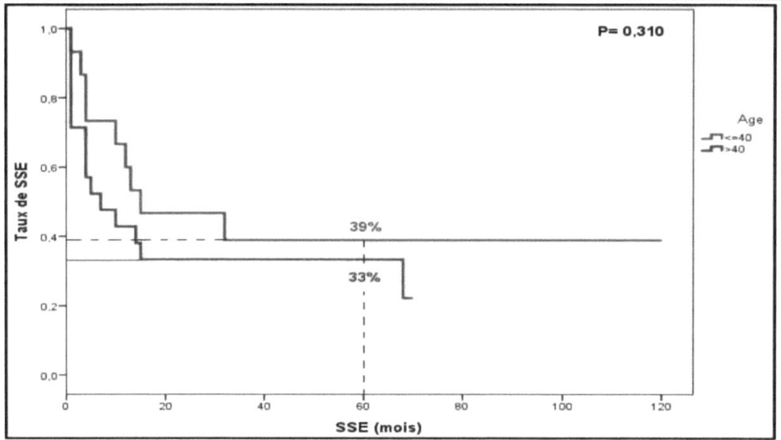

Figure 30: SES as a function of age.

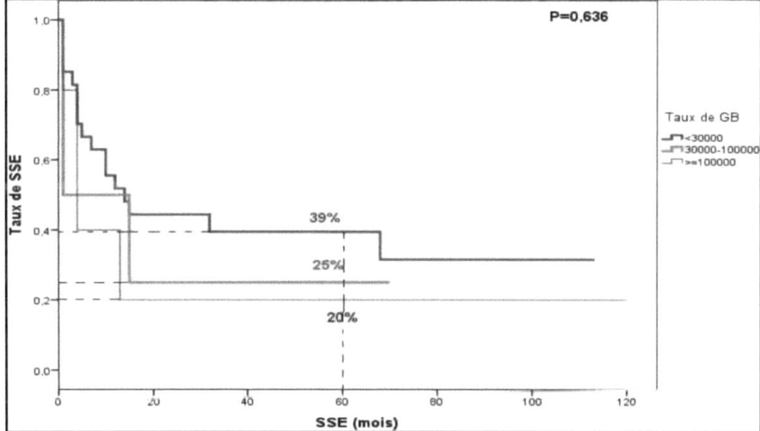

Figure 31: SES as a function of GB rate.

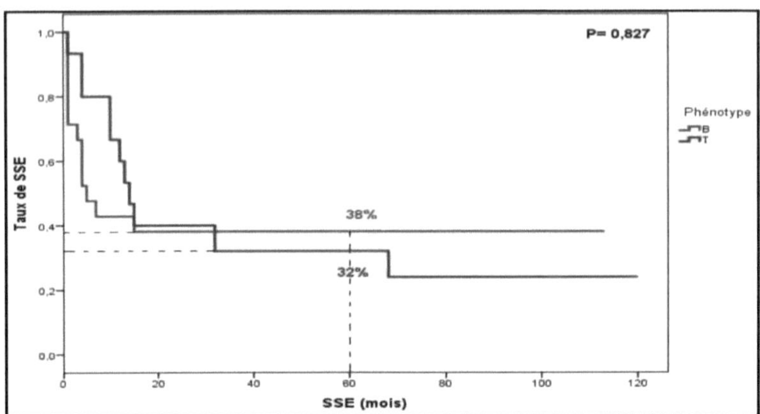

Figure 32: SES as a function of phenotype.

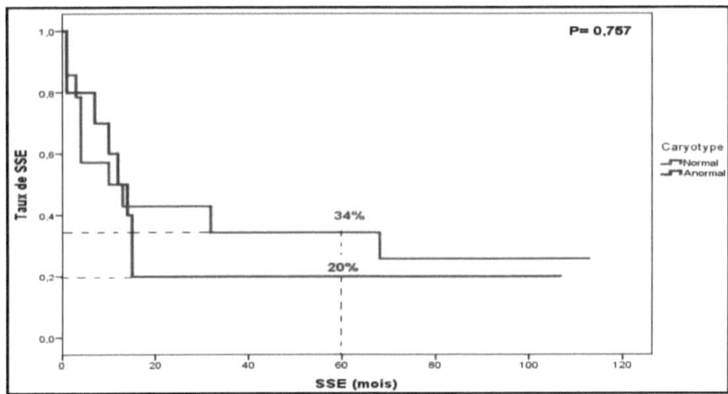

Figure 33: SES as a function of karyotype.

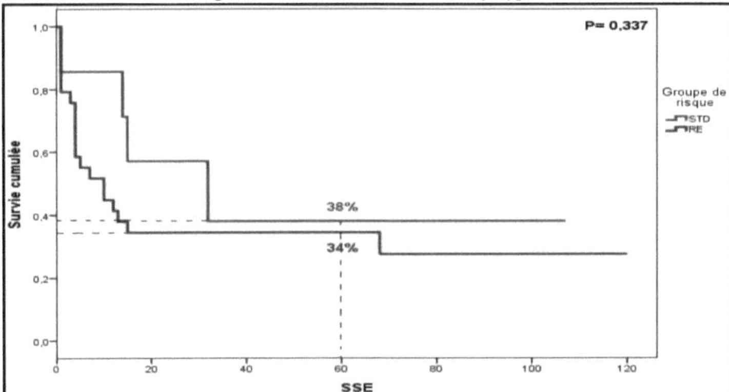

Figure 34: SES as a function of risk group.

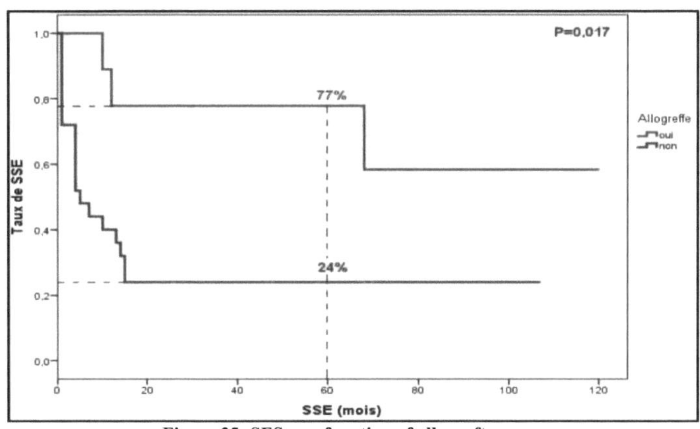

Figure 35: SES as a function of allograft group.

4.3 Therapeutic results in phi+ ALL

4.3.1 *Study of complete remission*

Seven patients (70%) had CR after 1 course of chemotherapy and two patients had CR after 2 courses, giving an overall CR rate of 90%.

One patient (10%) had failed after 2 courses of chemotherapy (induction and consolidation) and died of respiratory distress secondary to hypoxemic pneumonitis during salvage treatment.

The characteristics of patients who failed the induction treatment are detailed in Table XX.

Table XX: Characteristics of patients who failed after induction.

Age (years)	Gender	Tumour sd	GB G/L	Karyotype	Type of transcript	Start ttt ITK	Catch-up	RC	Cause of death
35	M	Yes	75,3	t(9,22) structural abnormalities of the Y chromosome	b3a2	D18 Induction (Imatinib)	Aracytin + novantrone + Imatinib	No	Hypoxemic lung disease
35	F	Yes	33,4	NI	e1a2	D8 Induction (Imatinib)	Consolidation	Yes	-
20	F	Yes	96,7	t(9,22) del 5q monosomy 7	e1a2	D8 Induction (Imatinib)	Consolidation	Yes	-

> Study of factors influencing CR

No factor significantly influenced the occurrence of CR. Sex and type of transcript appear to influence the occurrence of CR without the difference being significant (table XXI).

Table XXI: Study of factors influencing CR.

		RC	P Univariee
Age	<40 years (n=6) >40 years (n=4)	5 (83) 4(100)	1
Gender	Male (n=3) Female (n=7)	2 (67) 7(100)	0,300

Tumour syndrome	Yes (n=7) No (n=3)	6 (68) 3(100)	1
GB	<30000(n=6) >30000(n=4)	6(100) 3 (75)	0,400
Type of transcript	e1a2 (n=7) other (n=2)	7(100) 1 (50)	0,222

4.3.2 ***Study of relapses :***

Three patients (33%) of the nine in CR had a medullary relapse during the study period. The characteristics of relapsed patients are detailed in Table XXII.

Table XXII: Characteristics of patients who relapsed.

Age (years)	Gender	GB G/L	Karyotype	Transcribed type	Type ITK	Induction response	Allograft	Relapse time /RC	ttt relapse	Answer	State NMS
45	F	28	NI	e1a2	Imatinib D8 induction	RC (1cure)	No donor	8 months	Yes	Failure	DCD
20	F	96	t(9,22) monos 7 Del 5q	e1a2	Imatinib D8 induction	RC (2 treatments)	Refusal	8 months	No	-	DCD
32	F	11	NI	e1a2	Imatinib D10 induction	RC (1cure)	No POS	7 months	Yes	RC	VV

> Study of factors influencing relapse

No factor significantly influenced relapse in our series (table XXIII).

Table XXIII: Factors influencing relapse.

		Relapse (%)	P in univariee
Age	<40 years (n=5) >40 years (n=4)	2 (40) 1 (25)	1
Gender	Male (n=2) Female (n=7)	0 3 (43)	0,500
Tumour syndrome	Yes (n=6) No (n=3)	3 (50) 0	0,464
GB	<30000/mm^3 (n=6) >30000/mm^3 (n=3)	2 (33) 1 (33)	1
RC 1 cure	yes (n=7) no (n=2)	2 (29) 1 (50)	1
Allograft	yes (n=4) no (n=4)	0 2 (50)	0,429

4.3.3 ***Study of deaths:***

Among the 10 patients treated, there were 5 deaths in our series (50%) (Table XXIV):

- 3 patients died as a result of disease progression (one failed and two relapsed)
- One patient died during consolidation treatment due to septic shock.
- One patient died post allograft from CMV reactivation.

Table XXIV: Characteristics of decedent patients.

Age	Gender	GB G/L	Karyotype	Transcribed type	ITK	Induction response	Phase ttt	Bcr Abl ratio	Cause of death
50	M	24	Failure	e1a2	Imatinib J26 induction	RC (1cure)	C4 Hyper CVAD	Undetectable 10^{-4}	EDC Septic
45	F	28,2	Failure	e1a2	Imatinib D1 induction	RC (1cure)	Dexa + imatinib	0,62%	Evolution of the disease
44	F	6,1	Failure	e1a2	Imatinib 2eme cure	RC (2 treatments)	3 months post allograft	0,001 %	GVH+ CMV
20	F	96,7	T (9,22) + del 5q monosomy7	e1a2	Imatinib D8 induction	RC (2 treatments)	C7 Hyper CVAD	31%	Evolution of the disease
35	M	75,3	T (9,22) + structural abnormalities of the Y chromosome	b3a2	Imatinib J18 induction	Failure	Catch-up aracytin novantrone	-	Hypoxemic lung disease

4.3.4 ***Allogeneic bone marrow transplants***

Among the 9 patients in CR :

- Eight were indicated for allogeneic transplantation (9eme were aged > 50).
- Seven had an HLA-matched donor.
- Four were allografted in RC1: 2 refused grafts and one patient relapsed before allografting.

The median time to allograft in our series was 10 weeks after complete remission (extreme 8-16 weeks).

Of the 3 patients who relapsed, two received salvage treatment, one of whom underwent 2eme CR and allograft.

The feasibility and outcome of allografting are detailed in figure 36.

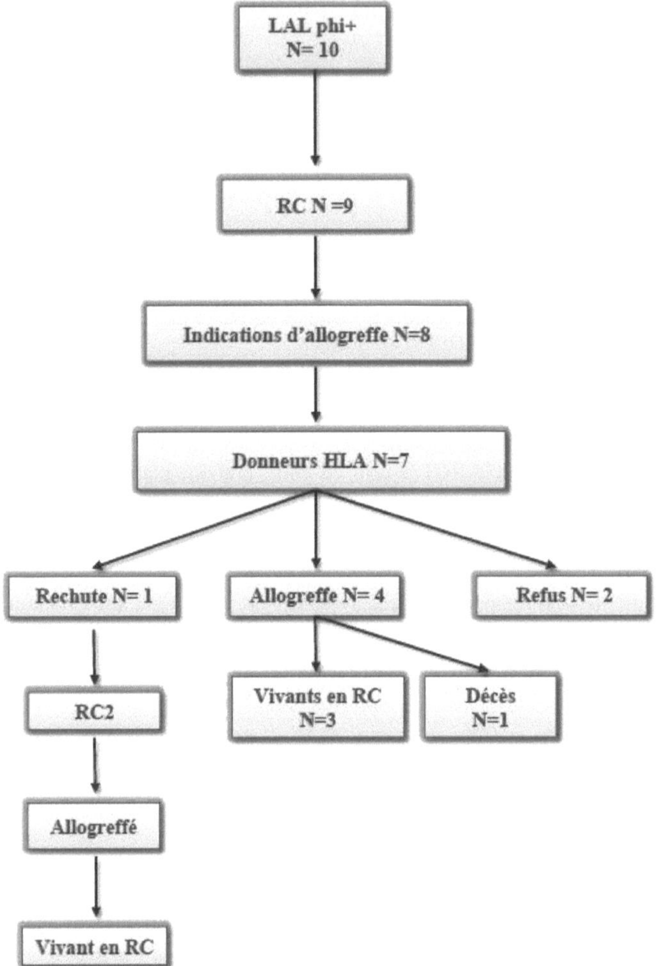

Figure 36: Bone marrow allograft in phi+ ALL patients.

4.3.5 ***Molecular monitoring of phi+ ALL patients in CR***

Of the nine CR patients, seven had molecular monitoring of residual disease using PCR.

Three patients had molecular failure and were indicated for switch to 2eme generation TKIs, which was carried out in 2 cases (management problem for the 3).^{eme}

Table XXV below details the molecular follow-up of phi+ ALL patients undergoing CR.

Table XXV: Molecular monitoring of phi+ ALL patients undergoing CR.

Year	Age (years)	Type of transcript	Type ITK	MRD				Switch ITK	State NMS	MRD DDN (%)
				Induction (%)	3 months (%)	6 months (%)	12 months (%)			
2014	**20**	e1a2	ITK1	100	20	5	31	No	Death and illness	31
2014	**44**	e1a2	ITK1	80	0,5	-	-	No	Post-transplant death	0,001
2015	**35**	e1a2	ITK1	71	-	7	-	Yes dasatinib	RC	RMC
2011	**53**	b2a2	ITK1	2	0,5	0 ,17	1,2	Yes dasatinib	RC	RM4
2015	**35**	e1a2	ITK1	1,5	0,01	-	-	No	RC	
2014	**50**	e1a2	ITK1	1	Undetectable 10^{-4}	-	-	No	Septic tank	Undetectable 10^{-4}
2011	**45**	e1a2	ITK1	Positive	-	0,009		No	Death and illness	0,62
2010	**32**	e1a2	ITK1	Negative*	-	-	-	No	RC	-
2011	**38**	Negative	ITK1	-	-	-	-	No	RC	-

*Molecular biology was carried out using a qualitative method.

4.3.6 ***Survival study :***

4.3.6.1 ***Overall survival :***

For a median follow-up of 57 months, the overall survival rate for the entire population was 60% at 1 year and 50% at both 2 and 5 years (Figure 37).

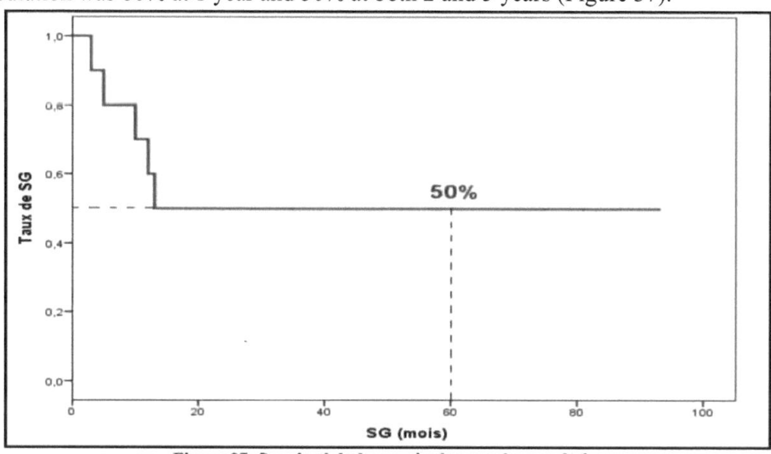

Figure 37: Survie globale au sein de toute la population.

> ***Study of factors influencing overall survival :***

No factor had a statistically significant influence on OS in our series in univariate analysis. However, age < 40 years and allogeneic bone marrow transplantation were correlated with better OS without the difference being significant. (Table XXVI).

Table XXVI: Factors influencing OS.

		% overall survival at 5 years	**P Univariee**
Age	<40 years	66	
	>40 years	25	0, 198
Gender	Male Female	33	
		57	0,229
Tumour syndrome	Yes	57	
	No	33	0,390
GB	<30000/mm^3	50	
	>30000/mm^3	50	0,973
Allograft	Yes	80	0,145
	No	20	

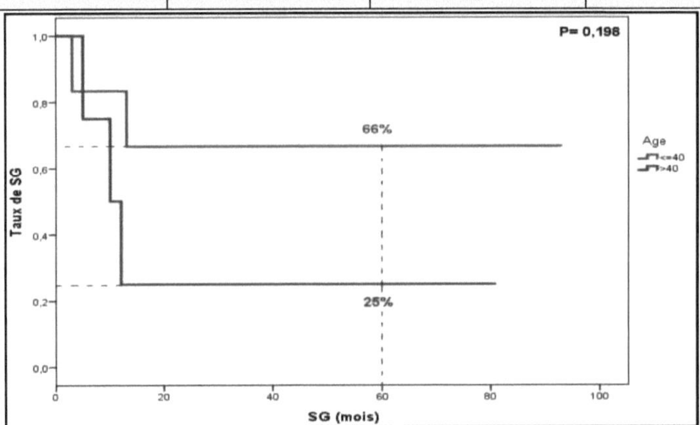

Figure 38: Overall survival as a function of Page.

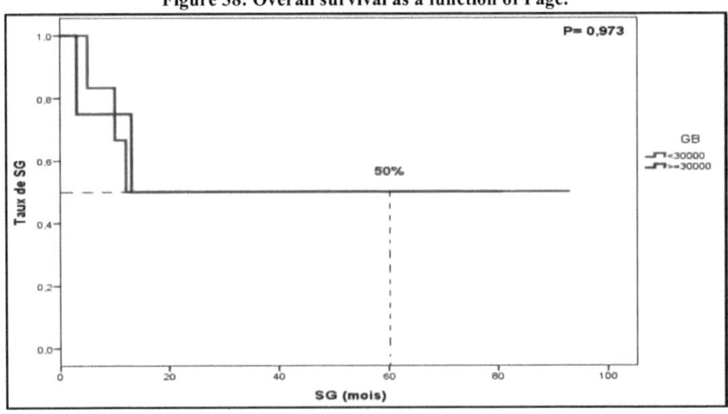

Figure 39: Overall survival as a function of white blood cell count.

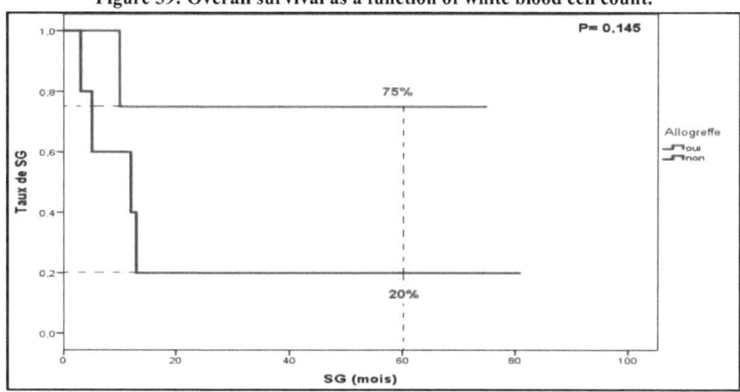

Figure 40: Overall survival as a function of allograft rate.

4.3.6.2 *Relapse-free survival*

The SRH was 58% at 1, 2 and 5 years (Figure 41).

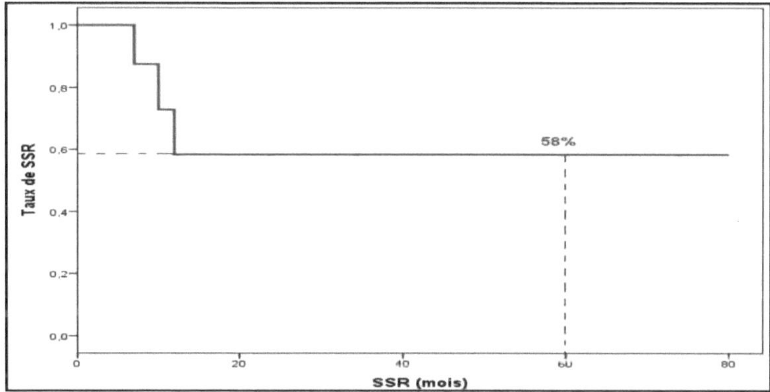

Figure 41: Relapse-free survival.

> ***Study of the factors influencing SRH :***

No factor had a statistically significant influence on SRH in our series. Allogeneic bone marrow transplantation and the absence of a tumour syndrome appear to be factors influencing SRH but not significantly (p=0.394 and 0.377 respectively).

The factors influencing SSR are detailed in table XXVII.

Table XXVII: Factors influencing SSR.

		% SSR at 5 years	P
Age	<40 years	60	0,907
	>40 years	50	
Tumour syndrome	Yes	50	
	No	100	0,377
GB	<30000/mm^3	53	0,577
	>=30000/mm^3	66	
Allograft	Yes	80	0,116
	No	33	

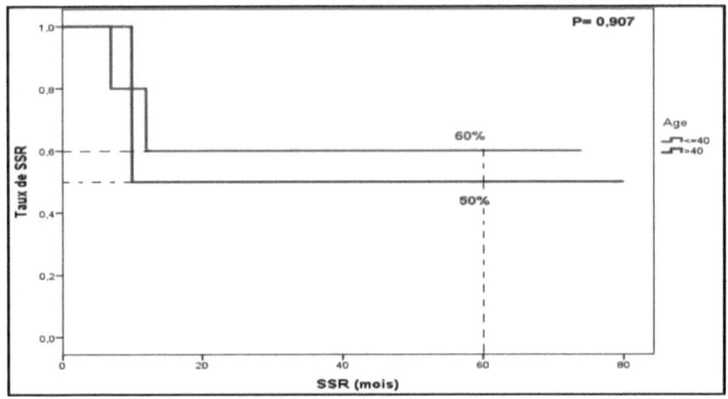

Figure 42: SSR by age.

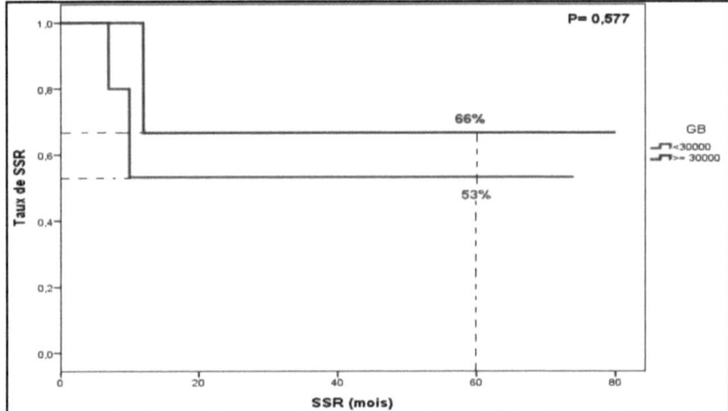

Figure 43: SSR as a function of white blood cell count.

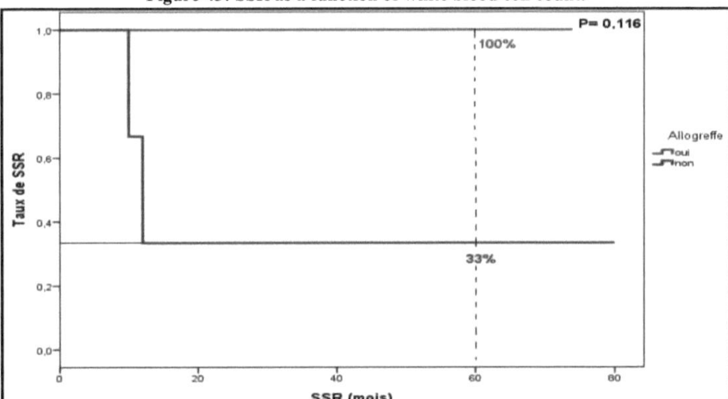

Figure 44: SSR according to allograft.

4.3.6.3 *Event-free survival:*

The SES was 40% at 1, 2 and 5 years (Figure 45).

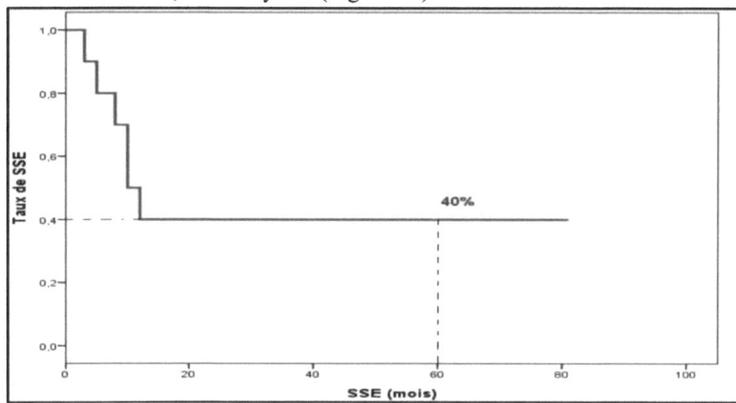

Figure 45: SES within the entire population.

> ***Study of the factors influencing SES :***

No factor significantly influenced SES in our series. Allogeneic bone marrow transplantation appeared to be a factor influencing SES, but not significantly (p=0.115).

The factors influencing SES are detailed in Table XXVIII.

Table XXVIII: Factors influencing SES.

		% SSE is 5 years old	P
Age	<40 years	50	0,524
	>40 years	25	
Gender		33	0,349
	Male Female	42	
Tumour syndrome	Yes	42	0,744
	No	33	
GB	$<30000/mm^3$	33	0,626
	$>30000/mm^3$	50	
Allograft	Yes	75	0,115
	No	20	

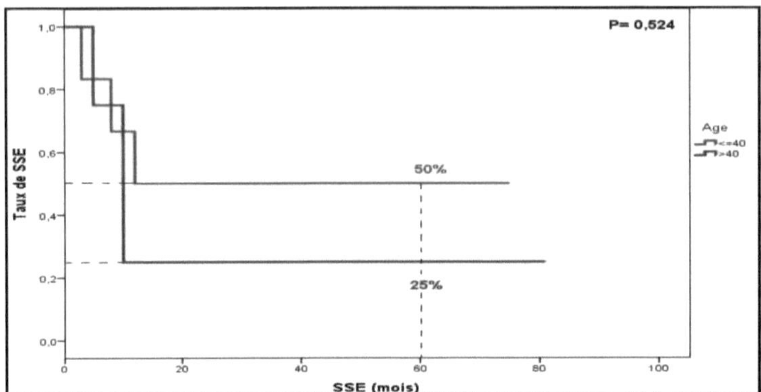

Figure 46: SES as a function of age.

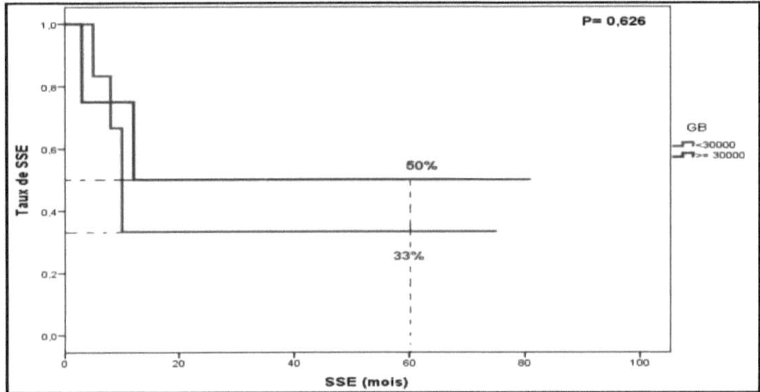

Figure 47: SES as a function of white blood cell count.

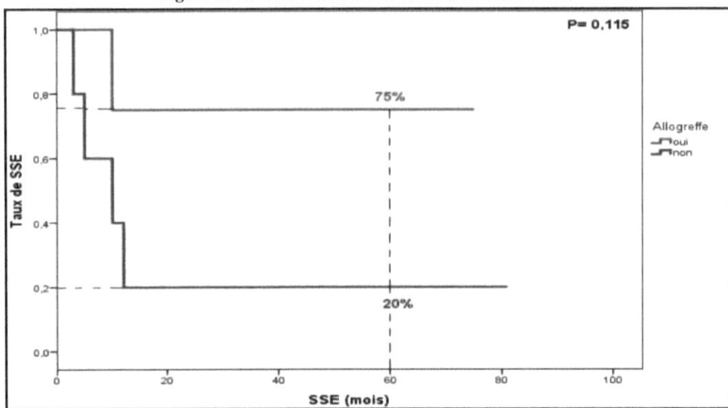

Figure 48: SES as a function of allograft.

4.4 Toxicity of treatment

It is graded according to the World Health Organisation (WHO) classification (Appendix 4).

4.4.1 *Non-phi+ LALs*

> ***Hematological toxicity during induction treatment***

The most frequent hematological toxicity was neutropenia followed by anaemia and thrombocytopenia (Table XXIX).

Table XXIX: Hematological toxicity during induction treatment of non-phi+ ALL.

Hematological toxicity	Grade III or IV in
Anemie	70
Thrombocytopenia	64
Neutropenia	79

> ***Infectious toxicity***

1) <u>During the induction treatment</u>

Febrile neutropenia was noted in 31 cases. An infectious site was found in 15 cases: digestive in 5 cases, cutaneous in 3 cases, urinary in 2 cases, anal in 2 cases, pulmonary in 1 case, a thyroid abscess in 1 case and ENT in 1 case. Septicemia was noted in 10 cases, i.e. 27% of cases. The most frequent germs were :

S Staphylococcus aureus (2 cases).

S Klebsiella pneumoniae (2 cases).

S Stenetrophomonas maltophilia (2 cases).

S Acinetobacter baumani (1 case).

S Achromobacter xylosoxi (1 case).

S Klebsiella oxytoca (1 case).

S Enterobacter cloacae (1 case).

Pulmonary aspergillosis was considered in 5 cases (13% of cases). It was probable in 3 cases and possible in 2.

2) <u>During post-induction treatment</u>

Febrile neutropenia was noted in 26 cases. An infectious site was found in 18 cases, of the following types: digestive in 6 cases, pulmonary in 3 cases, urinary in 2 cases, anal in 1 case, mucositis in 3 cases, dental in 1 case and ENT in 2 cases. Septicemia with klepsial pneumonia was noted in 1 case.

> ***Metabolic toxicity***

1) <u>During the induction treatment</u>

Cortico-induced diabetes was noted in 14 cases (38%), with acidotic coma in one case. Two cases of pancreatitis at 1'ASPA were noted, one of which was favourable.

Six cases (16%) presented a disturbance of the liver balance, such as cytolysis associated with ASPA, with a favourable outcome.

2) <u>Post-induction treatment</u>

S Diabetes disequilibrium was noted in 2 cases.

S Acute organic renal failure secondary to MTX in 1 case.

S Hepatic cytolysis was noted in 3 cases.
S Icterus secondary to the administration of Purinethol in one case.

> ***Other toxicities***

1) ***<u>During the induction treatment</u>***

Cerebral thrombophlebitis was noted in three of our patients, i.e. 7% of cases, the origin of which was related to the administration of ASPA.

A sub-occlusive syndrome secondary to the administration of Oncovin in one case.

2) ***<u>Post-induction treatment</u>***

S Allergic reaction to ASPA = 7 cases.
S Allergic reaction to Erwiniase = 1 case.
S Folinic acid shock = 1 case.
S Subacute extradural haematoma = 1 case.
S Extravasation of chemotherapy product = 1 case.

4.4.2 ***phi+ LAL***

> ***Hematological toxicity during induction treatment***

Details of hematological toxicity during induction treatment are given in table XXX.

Table XXX: Hematological toxicity during induction treatment of phi+ ALL.

Hematological toxicity	Grade III or IV in
Anemie	80
Thrombocytopenia	80
Neutropenia	90

> ***Infectious toxicity***

1) ***<u>During the induction treatment</u>***

Febrile neutropenia was noted in all 10 cases. The portal of entry was anal in 4 cases, ENT in 1 case (angina), cutaneous in 1 case (panaris) and mucosal in 1 case (oral candidiasis). Pulmonary aspergillosis was noted in 2 cases (possible in 1 case and probable in 1 case).

In 4 cases, no infectious outbreaks were found (table XXXI).

Table XXXI: Breakdown of febrile episodes by household.

Foyer		Number of cases
Anal	Crack	3
	Abces	1
ENT		1
Cutane		1
Mucous membrane		1
Pulmonary		2
Without fireplaces		4

2) ***<u>During post-induction treatment</u>***

6) cases of septicemia have been reported. The isolated germs are :

S Staphylococcus aureus: 1 case (with secondary pulmonary and splenic localisation).
S White staphylococcus: 1 case.

S Stenotrophomonas maltophilia: 2 cases.
S Klebsielle pneumoniae: 1 case.
S Enterobacter cloacae: 1 case.
Septic shock was noted in 3 cases. The outcome was favourable in two cases and death was noted in one.
Possible pulmonary aspergillosis was noted in 1 case.

> ***Metabolic toxicity***

Cortico-induced diabetes was noted in 3 cases during the induction treatment (30%). Of these 3, only one patient showed a loss of control of his diabetes during the consolidation treatments.
One patient developed acute organic renal failure secondary to MTX toxicity during consolidation treatments.
One patient presented with severe hypokalaemia (profuse diarrhoea).
Hepatic cytolysis was noted in 4 cases: 2 during induction treatment and 2 during consolidation treatment.

> ***Other toxicities***

Only one patient experienced an allergic reaction to Imatinib, consisting of facial flushing and vomiting. Subsequent reintroduction of Imatinib with premedication was uneventful.
Thrombophlebitis of the left lower limb secondary to oestroprogestins was noted in one case.

4 Discussion

1 Diagnostic aspect

1.1 Epidemiological data

1.1.1 *Frequency*

ALL has an overall incidence of 1 to 1.5 per 100,000 people (10). The peak incidence is between 4 and 5 years of age (4 to 5 cases per 100,000 people), with another peak at the age of 50 (2 cases per 100,000 people). ALL is the most common childhood leukaemia, but accounts for only 20% of adult leukaemias (11). ALL is rare in adults, with approximately 10,000 new cases diagnosed in Europe each year (12) (Figure 49).

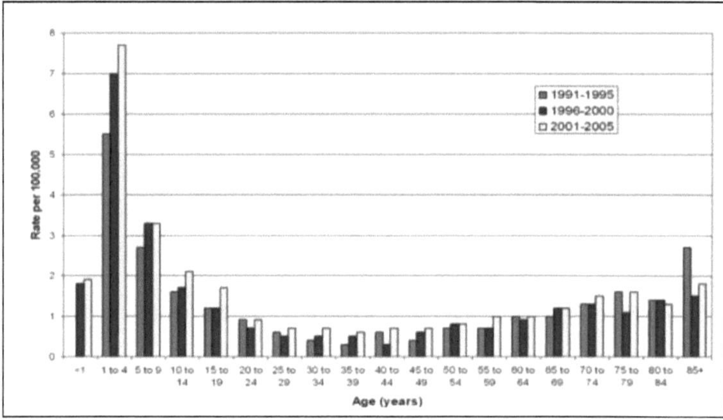

Figure 49 : Specific incidence rate of ALL by period of observation (13).

In an old study carried out in Sfax on 531 cases of leukaemia <iiguc\ the frequency of adult ALL was 19% of acute adult leukaemias and 12% of all acute leukaemias (14) (Figure 50).

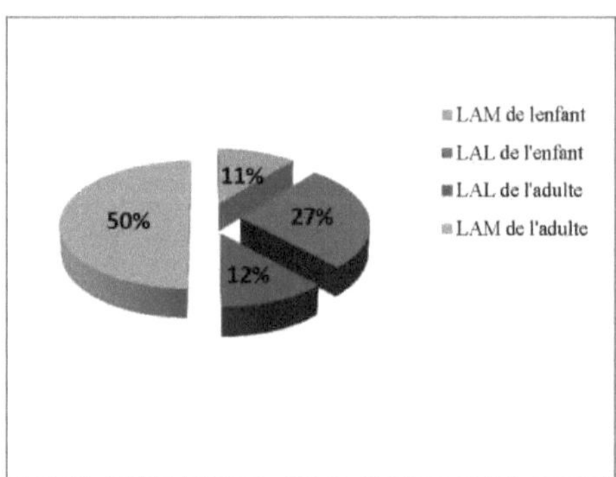

Figure 50: Frequency of each type of LA in Sfax (14).

1.1.2 *Geographical origin:*

A higher frequency of adult ALL was observed in the Sfax region, around 40% of cases, followed by the Sidi Bouzid, Gabes and Gafsa regions (18, 12 and 10% of cases respectively). These rates are slightly different from the previous local series, with a higher frequency in the Sidi Bouzid and Gabes regions (10 and 9% respectively) and a lower frequency in the Sfax and Gafsa regions (50 and 16% respectively) (7).

1.1.3 *Gender :*

A female predominance has been noted in our series for phi+ ALL and a slight male predominance for non-phi+ ALL. In various series in the literature, a male predominance has been described for both phi+ and non Ph+ ALL (15-18).

1.1.4 *Age :*

The median age in our series was 42 years with extremes ranging from 20 to 56 years: it was 42 years (extreme 27- 56 years) for non-phi+ ALL patients and 38 years (extreme 20- 55 years) for phi+ ALL patients.

This median age was higher than that described in the literature (27.5 to 38 years) (15-22) due to the fact that since 2009 we have been using the paediatric protocol for the treatment of adolescent and young adult ALL (up to 30 years) (Table XXXII).

Table XXXII: Median age of the different series in the literature.

Study group	Therapeutic Protocol	Year of study	Number of patients	Age group (years)	Median age (years)
Tunisia	**Our GRAALL/GRAAPH series**	2004- 2015	49	20- 56	42
	Hdiji (8) **LALA 94 (multi-centric)**	1997-2001	52	21-53	33
	Nasf (7) **LALA76, 78 and HPS 89**	1987-1996	58	16-90	42
	Bouallegue (23) **Hyper CVAD**	2003-2010	30	17-58	28
	Ben Neji (24) **GRAALL 2005**	2009-2012	22	25-45	37,5
France	***Thomas*** (16) **LALA 94**	1994-2002	922	15-55	33
	Huguet (15) **GRAALL 2003**	2003-2005	225	15-60	31
	Huguet (22) **GRAALL 2005**	2006-2014	787	18-59	36,1
Italy	***Annino*** (17) **GIMEMA**	1988-1994	794	12-60	27,5
	Bassan (19) **NILG ALL 09/00**	2009	280	16-66	38
Chicago	***Larson*** (18) **CALGB**	1991-1993	198	16-83	35
Spain	***Ribera*** (21) **PETHEMA**	1993-2002	222	15-50	27
Germany	***Gokbuget*** (20) **GMALL**	-	713	15-55	34
Brazil	***Wellington*** (25) **GMALL**	2009-2015	59	16-71	35
Emirates	***Hassan*** (26) **UKALL XII/ECOG E2993**	2000-2009	99	15-62	28

1.2 Clinical data

1.2.1 *Tumour syndrome*

A tumour syndrome was noted in 63% of cases, comparable to the former local series (67%) and less frequent than the Sousse series (96.6%) (7,23).

1.2.2 *Testicular damage*

Testicular involvement, which is classic in young boys, is exceptional in adults (4). In our series, no testicular involvement was noted.

1.2.3 *Damage to the central nervous system:*

In our series, central nervous system involvement was noted in 3 patients (5%), comparable to that described in the Sousse series (6.6%) (23) and in various series in the literature (5 to 10%) (6,11,26,27).

1.3 Biological data

1.3.1 *Hemogram*

The median WBC level in our series (10 G/L) was close to that in the literature (7.7 G/L to 16.8 G/L) (15-18,20,27) but lower than in the previous local series (7) and the Sousse series (23). Hyperleukocytosis >100 G/L was found in 12% of our cases, slightly less than in the previous local series and the Sousse series (34% and 24% respectively) (Table XXXIII).

Table XXXIII: Median GB rate for different series in the literature.

Study group	Therapeutic Protocol	Year of study	Number of patients	Median WBC rate (G/L)	GB> 100 G/L (%)
Tunisia	**Our GRAALL/GRAAPH series**	2004- 2015	49	10	6 (12)
	Nasfi (7) **LALA76, 78 and HPS 89**	1987-1996	58	97,3	19 (34)
	Bouallegue (23) **Hyper CVAD**	2003-2010	30	90,9	7 (24)
	Ben Neji (24) **GRAALL 2005**	2009-2012	22	14	-
France	***Thomas*** (16) **LALA 94**	1994-2002	922	14,4	-
	Huguet (15) **GRAALL 2003**	2003-2005	225	11,8	-
Italy	***Annino*** (17) **GIMEMA**	1988-1994	794	13,6	111(14)
	Bassan (19) **NILG ALL 09/00**	2009	280	16,5	-
Chicago	***Larson*** (18) **CALGB**	1991-1993	198	16,8	-
Brazil	***Wellington*** (25) **GMALL**	2009-2015	59	12,6	-
Chicago	***Kantarjian*** (27) **Hyper CVAD**	1992-1998.	204	7,7	-

1.3.2 *Immunophenotyping study*

In our series, the frequency of ALL B (65%) was comparable to the various series in the literature (varying between 60 and 79%) (15-18,22). However, the rate of B phenotype was higher than in the Sousse and Tunis series (23,24) (Table XXXIV). The phi+ ALLs were all of B phenotype both in our series and in the various series in the literature (25,26).

Table XXXIV: Phenotypic distribution of ALL from different series in the literature.

Serie	LALB (%)	LALT (%)	Biphenotypic (%)	Indifferencie (%)
Our GRAALL/GRAAPH series	32 (65)	16 (33)	1 (2)	-
***Hdiji* (8) LALA 94**	27 (60)	17 (37,8)	-	-
***Ben Neji* (24) GRAALL 2005**	9 (41)	13 (59)	-	-
***Bouallegue* (23) Hyper CVAD**	9 (39,1)	13 (41,9)	-	1 (3,2)
***Thomas* (16) LALA 94**	647 (72)	239 (26)	-	16 (2)
***Huguet* (15) GRAALL 2003**	149 (66)	76 (34)	-	-
***Huguet* (22) GRAALL 2005**	525(67)	262 (33)	-	-
***Annino* (17) GIMEMA**	513 (73)	154 (22)	-	39 (6)
***Larson* (18) CALGB**	116(79)	30 (21)	-	-

1.3.3 *Cytogenetic study*

Cytogenetic analysis in ALL has become an essential part of the diagnosis prior to the initiation of treatment. The clonal chromosomal abnormalities found have an independent prognostic value, which makes karyotyping essential, as it conditions therapy.

The classification of ALL proposed by the WHO in 2008 and revised in 2016 reflects this dimension (28).

> *Conventional cytogenetics:* This detects clonal chromosomal abnormalities in 70% to 84% of adults with ALL (29,30). In our series, this study detected cytogenetic abnormalities in 51% of cases, slightly more than the Sousse series (31% of cases) (23).

Some of these anomalies have a good prognosis, such as hyperdiploidy detected in 3% of cases, less frequent than the Sousse series (10%) (23). Other anomalies have a poor prognosis such as translocation (9,22), found in 18% of cases, more frequent than the Sousse series (3%) (23) and close to the different series in the literature (16,19). The t (4,11), not found in our series, is reported in 4 to 9% of cases and is associated with a poor prognosis (15,16,31).

> *Fluorescent in situ hybridization or FISH:* This completes the conventional karyotype. Three main types of probe are used in haematological cytogenetics: centromeric probes or probes of the long arm of the Y and locus-specific or single-sequence probes which reveal cryptic structural anomalies such as insertions of

sequences of too small a size which escape conventional karyotyping.

The main cytogenetic abnormalities described in the literature in B and T ALL are detailed in tables XXXV, XXXVI and XXXVII (32).

Table XXXV: Cytogenetic abnormalities in ALL (32).

LAL	Anomaly	Incidence	Prognosis	Specific treatment?
B+T	Hyperdiploidy	< 10% in adults/30-35 X in children	Favourable	
	Hypodiploid, haploid and quasi-tnploid forms	< 5% in adults	Unfavourable	
	MIL storage compartments	80% in children under 1 year of age, exceptional above this age in children, 10% in adults.		Demethylating agents, UK. FLT3 inhibitors, new nucleoside analogues Iclofar abrne)
	Complex karyotypes (> 5 anomalies)	< 5% in adults		

Table XXXVI: Cytogenetic abnormalities in B-ALL (32).

LAL	Anoma lie	Incidence	Prognosis	Specific treatment?
B	tt9;22Xq34;q 1D/BCRABL1	30-40% in adults/<5% in Γchildren	Unfavourable	ITK
	FCF3-PBX1 and *TCF3HLF*	4% of childhood and young adult ALL		
	(IAMP21)	Mainly children and teenagers		
	Mutations/deletions in the *IKZF1* gene	~ ya LAL Ph*, 1/3 LAL non Ph+/15% of LAL B of (child)		
	LAL BCR-ABL1 like	15% of childhood ALL. and probably a significant proportion in the 15-25 age group		ΓΓK. *JAK2* inhibitors, *FLT3* inhibitors, Rapamycin
	CRLF2 storage compartments	50% of Down syndrome-associated ALL and up to 50% of BCR-ABL1 Ake ALL		
	PAX5 mutation	Early in leukemogenesis B about 30% of ALL B	?	
	K12;21Kpl2;q22)/TELAMLI	1-3% in adults/25% in children	Favourable	
	Intragenic deletion of ERG	■/3%		

Table XXXVII: Cytogenetic abnormalities in T-ALL (32).

LAL	Anoma lie	Incidence	Prognosis	Specific treatment?
T	Overexpression *of TALI* -t(l ;14) (p32 ;ql 1) SL-TAL for example.	SIL TAL = 20% of childhood T-ALL with t(l:14)		
	K5;14) /surexpression of *TLX3/H0X11L2*	10-15% in adults		
	ttlO :ll)(pl3 ;ql4) with creation of the CALM-AF10 fusion gene	7% of T-ALL but > 30% of immature T-ALL		
	Mutations in RAS or PTEN	20-25%		
	Overexpression of *BAALC*		. Unfavourable	
	JAK1/2 mutations. *PTPN2*, IL7-R			JAK inhibitors
	FLT3 mutations	24%		ITK. FLT3 inhibitors
	ETP. especially if CALM-AF10+.	8%		
	Loss of function (allelic loss, deletion or epigenetic regulation) of tumour suppressor genes (e.g. *CDKN2A/B)*			
	t(10;14), t(7;101/expression of *TLX1/HOXU*	10-20% in adults	Favourable	
	Mutations in *NOTCH1* or FBXW7	>60%		

1.3.4 *Molecular biology:*

It allows the identification of fusion transcripts, molecular equivalents of certain chromosomal translocations (table XXXVIII). It has a prognostic value but is also of major interest in the evaluation of residual disease and may be used in the subsequent indication for bone marrow allograft transplantation (33).

Only the Bcr-Abl transcript, the molecular equivalent of t(9,22) (q34, q11), was detected in our series. It was positive in 10 cases, whereas in only one case did we find t(9,22) with a negative transcript. At the Institut Pasteur in Tunis, only the most frequent Bcr-Abl transcripts are detected; a rare transcript could not be detected.

In conclusion, the frequency of phi+ ALL was therefore 22%, comparable with the various series in the literature varying between 15 and 30% (15,16,26,34) and reaching 50% in the oldest patients (35).

Depending on the breakpoint in the BCR gene, 2 types of protein may be formed:

either p190 or p210. The former is seen exclusively in phi+ ALL, whereas the p210 protein is found in only 20-40% of cases (36). In our series, the transcript type was p190 in 70% of cases and p210 in 30%.

Table XXXVIII: The main cytogenetic abnormalities and their molecular rearrangements (6).

Cytogenetic abnormalities	Frequency (%)	Genes
t(9,22) (q34, q11)	15-25	BCR-ABL
del(11) (q21-23)	25-30	ATM
del (17,19)	<5	E2A-HLF
t(4,11), t(9,11)	5-10	MLL
t(7,9) (q34-q32)	<1	TAL2
t(1 ;19)	<5	E2A-PBX1
t(10 ;14)	5-10	HOX11

2 Therapeutic results :

2.1 Non-phi+ LAL :

2.1.1 *Pre-phase response:*

Corticosensitivity was initially shown to be a good prognostic factor in children, and this notion has since been extended to adult protocols. It was first tested by *Annino*, who showed that corticosensitivity is an important prognostic factor in the treatment of adult ALL, with better survival in the corticosensitive group (17). Corticosensitivity was found in 89% of our series, comparable to the various series in the literature (15,17,24) (Table XXXIX). Predictors of corticoresistance were age and hyperleukocytic forms, both in our series and in the literature (17). In our series, a WBC count < 10,000/mm^3 significantly influenced corticosensitivity (p=0.04).

Table XXXIX: Corticosensitivity according to series.

Serie	Protocol	Corticosensitivity
Our series **Sfax**	Tunisian GRAALL 2003 and 2005	89%
Ben Neji (24) **GRAALL 2005**	GRAALL2005	79%
Annino **(17) Italy**	GIMEMMA ALL 0288	66%
Huguet **(15) France**	GRAALL 2003	75%

2.1.2 *Chemosensitivity :*

Chemosensitivity was noted in 83% of cases, comparable to various series in the literature (15). Chemosensitivity at D15 is correlated with a good prognosis (37).

2.1.3 *Study of complete remission:*

In our series, 90% of our patients were in CR after one induction treatment and 93% after two treatments. This rate is higher than the former local series and the Sousse series (86% and 76.6% respectively) (7,23) and comparable with different series in the literature (15-17,19,26) (Table XL).

Two patients (5%) had failed therapy after two courses of chemotherapy. This rate is lower than the former local series (14%) (7), comparable to the results of the Sousse series (6.6%) (23) and to different series in the literature (16,19,20,25,38). The following table summarises the CR and failure rates for adult ALL reported in the various literature series.

Table XL: CR and failure rates for different series in the literature.

Serie	Protocol	Number of patients	CR rate (%)	% induction failure
Our* Sfax *series	GRAALL 2003 and 2005	39	93	5
***Nasf* 1999(7) Sfax**	LALA 76, 87 and HPS 89	58	86	14
***Hdiji* 2013 (8) Tunisia (multicentre)**	LALA 94	45	69	9
***Ben Neji 2013*(24) Tunis**	GRAALL 2005	22	81	19
***Bouallegue* 2012 (23) Sousse**	H CVAD	30	76,6	3
***Thomas* 2004(16) F rance**	LALA 94	922	84	11
***Huguet* 2009(15) F rance**	GRAALL 2003	225	93,5	0,4
***Huguet* 2018 (22) F rance**	GRAALL 2005	787	91,9	-
***Annino* 2002(17) Italy**	GIMEMA ALL 0288	794	86	11
***Bassan* 2009(19) Italy**	NILG	236	84,3	7,5
***Gokbuget 2007*(20) Germany**	GMALL	713	89	6
***Hassan* 2012(26) Emirates**	UKALL XII/ ECOG E2993	99	85,7	13
***Stock* 2013 (34) Chicago**	CALGB 19802	163	80	10
***Kenneth* 2016 (38) Australia**	LAM Protocol	20	79	5
***Willington2018*(25) Brazil**	GMALL	59	76	6,8

2.1.4 *Stratification of patients according to risk group*

Several schemes for stratifying patients according to prognostic factors have been developed with the aim of adapting treatment and defining the group of patients eligible for intensified therapy by bone marrow allograft. The prognostic factors are divided into 4 groups:

> **Early parameters:** age, WBC level, initial CNS involvement, extra-medullary involvement.

> **Immunological phenotype:** Pro-B or pre-B CD10- ALL and T-ALL of precocious or mature phenotype are classified as high risk (39).

> **Cytogenetic and molecular abnormalities:** identified by the WHO classification (39,40).

> **Response to treatment**: corticosensitivity, chemosensitivity, CR and level of residual disease.

Concerning the evaluation of residual disease: several therapeutic groups have used MRD in prognostic classification with different thresholds: this threshold was 10^{-2} after induction and after the 3eme consolidation block (MRD1 and MRD2 respectively) in the GRAALL 2005 protocol, however it is not used either in prognostic classification or in the indication for allograft transplantation (22). More recently, in the GRAALL 2014 trial, MRD1 <10^{-3} is considered a high-risk factor, whereas MRD1 >10^{-3} or MRD2 >10-4 are considered very high-risk factors justifying Vindication of allograft in RC1 (41).

In our series, 80% of our patients are treated according to the RE group and 20% according to the STD group. The frequency of patients classified as high risk is higher than in the literature, ranging from 43 to 68% (15,16,25) (Table XLI).

Table XLI: Breakdown of risk groups according to literature series.

Serie	Protocol	STD	BR %
Our series **Sfax**	GRAALL 2003 and 2005	20	80
***Huguet* 2009(15) France**	GRAALL 2003	34	66
***Thomas* 2004(16) France**	LALA 94	59	33
***Willington2018*(25)** **Brazil**	GMALL	32	68

The following table shows the stratification of ALL in the different protocols reported in the literature (Table XLII).

Table XLII: Therapeutic stratification of ALL into risk groups.

Protocol	Standard risk	High risk
Our GRAALL 2003 series	Absence of ER criteria	* Only 1 of the following factors: - LALB with WBC>30,000/mm3. - ALL with WBC>100 000/mm3. - LAL pro B - Common LAL B. - Immature LALT. - 1 (4,11) or 11q23 anomaly. - Neuromeningitis. - Corticoresistance at D8. - Chemoresistance at D15. - No CR after induction treatment.
Our GRAALL 2005 series	Absence of ER criteria	In addition to the GRAALL 2003 criteria - All LALB -1 (1,19), hypo-diploidy, pres triploidy, complex karyotype (> 5 anomalies)
GRAALL 2003 (15)	Absence of ER criteria	*ALL B with WBC > 30 G/L at diagnosis. *Presence of neuromeningeal involvement. *Presence of t(4;11) and/or MLL-AF4, t(1; 19). and/or E2A-PBX1, hypoploidy and/or close to triploidy * Corticoresistance and/or chemoresistance. *No RC after induction, high MRD.
GRAALL 2005 (22)	Absence of ER criteria	In addition to the GRAALL 2003 criteria B-ALL with CD10 . Complex karyotype.
LALA-94 (16)	All ALL unless no CR after induction B-ALL with the following characteristics: *Absence of neuro-meningeal involvement	***Group 2*** No SR criteria with absence of Philadelphia chromosome and neuromeningeal involvement

	* Absence of Philadelphia chromosome, t(4;11), t(1;19) or 11q23 abnormalities * WBC count < 30 G/L at diagnosis *CD10/CD19, or CD20/CD19 and absence of myeloid markers *RC after a course of chemotherapy.	Failure or non-performance of immunophenotyping or cytogenetic tests. ***Group 3***: ALL with presence of Philadelphia chromosome and/or Bcr-abl +. ***Group 4***: ALL with neuromeningeal involvement.
MRC UKALL XII/ECOG E2993 (42)	Age < 35 obtaining a CR before 4 weeks. ALL B with WBC <30 G/L, ALL T with WBC <100 G/L.	Age > 35. Obtained a RC after 4 weeks. ALL B with WBC <30 G/L, ALL T with WBC >100 G/L.
HOVON (43)	No risk factors.	**One of the following criteria:** Presence of t (9;22), t (4;11) or t (1;19). Phenotype pro B. LAL B with WBC >30 G/L, LAL T with WBC >100 G/L. Achievement of late CR (after 4 weeks of induction treatment).

2.1.5 *Study of deaths:*

2.1.5.1 *Induction death :*

Although lower than the former local series (27%) and comparable to that of the Tunis series, the induction death rate in our series was higher than that of the Sousse series and the various series in the literature ranging from 4.1 to 17% (15-17,19,23,44) (table XLIII). This high rate of induction deaths could be explained by inadequate management during the aplasia period, either because of the absence of a sterile isolation unit (absence of laminar flow) or because of inadequate supportive treatment during the aplasia period.

Table XLIII: Percentage of induction deaths and relapses in the various literature series.

Serie	Protocol	Number of patients	% Induction	% Relapse
Our Sfax series	GRAALL 2003 and 2005	39	19	50
***Nasfi* 1999(7) Sfax**	LALA76, 87 and HPS 89	58	27	74
***Bouallegue2012* (23) Sousse**	H CVAD	30	6,6	39,1
***Ben Neji* (24) Tunis**	GRAALL 2005	22	18	50
***Thomas* 2004(16) France**	LALA 94	922	5	55
***Huguet* 2009(15) France**	GRAALL 2003	225	6	31
***Huguet* 2018 (22) France**	GRAALL 2005	787	5,6	29,8
***Annino* 2002(17) Italy**	GIMEMA ALL 0288	794	7	60
***Bassan* 2009(19) Italy**	NILG	236	8,2	49,6
***Hassan* 2012(26) Emirates**	UKALL XII/ ECOG E2993	99	4,1	-
***Stock* 2013(34) Chicago**	CALGB 19802	163	10	27
***Kenneth* 2016 (38) Australia**	LAM Protocol	20	11	40
***Willington* 2018 (25) Brazil**	GMALL	59	17	37

2.1.5.2 *Deaths on consolidation*

Three toxic deaths occurred during consolidation treatment (10%). This rate is lower than that of the Sousse series (53%) (23). Among our 3 deaths: one patient died during maintenance treatment due to septic shock and 2 patients died post allograft.

2.1.6 ***Relapse studies :***

2.1.6.1 ***Frequency :***

Although the CR rate for adult ALL is over 90%, only 30 to 40% of patients have prolonged SES (40). This rate is partly due to the high frequency of relapses, which constitute a major problem in the revolution of ALL. These relapses may be early or late, medullary and/or extra-medullary (neuromeningeal or testicular). Isolated medullary relapses are the most common.

In our series, 50% of our patients followed for ALL presented a relapse. This rate is lower than the previous local series (74%) (7) and comparable with the various series in the literature (16,17,19) (Table XLIII).

Among the relapses, 38% presented an isolated medullary relapse, 3% an isolated neuromeningeal relapse and 7% medullary and neuromeningeal relapse, these rates are comparable to those of the Sousse series (23). Compared with the former local series, there was a lower frequency of isolated medullary, isolated meningeal and testicular relapse (38 vs 52%, 3 vs 22% and 0 vs 4% respectively) (table XLIV).

The following table shows the frequency and location of relapses in our series and in other series in the literature:

Table XLIV: Location of relapse according to the different series.

	Relapse rate (%)	Medullary relapse (%)	Meningeal relapse (%)	Testicular relapse (%)	Medullary + meningeal relapse (%)	Medullary + testicular relapse (%)
Our series	50	38	3	-	7	-
***Nasfi* 1999(7)**	74	52	22	4	9	-
***Bouallague* 2012 (23)**	39,1	26	4,3	-	8,69	-
***Huguet* 2018 (22)**	29,8	76	9	-	8	-
***Kantarjian* 2000(27)**	45,9	17,9	14	-	4	-

2.1.6.2 ***Delay in onset of relapse***

Most relapses occur during the first two years after complete remission. They are early and all the more serious if they occur in the first year, and late if they occur after that. In our series, 71% of relapses occurred during the first 1ere years of CR and 93% of relapses occurred during the first 2 years. Our results are comparable to the previous local series (7) and to the series published by *Annino* (17).

2.1.6.3 ***Treatment of relapses***

The prognosis for relapse is poor. Despite a 2eme complete remission rate that varies between 20% and 83%, this RC2 is short-lived (45). The disease-free survival rate of relapsed patients treated with chemotherapy followed by allograft is only 7% to 24% (46).

There is no clear consensus on the 2eme line treatment of adult ALL. Treatment depends on the type of chemotherapy used in 1ere line, the duration of 1ere remission, age and whether or not allogeneic transplantation is used in 1ere line.

Several types of chemotherapy have been described in the literature: high-dose Aracytin-based regimens in combination with Antracycline, the FLAG protocol, H CVAD, Clofarabine-based chemotherapies (47-56) (Table XLV).

Table XLV: Salvage treatment for ALL.

Chemotherapy	Number of patients	RC2 rate	Allograft	SG
Aracytine 3g/m² D1-J5 + IDA 40mg/m² D3 (56)	135	55%	40%	6 months
Aracytine 3g/m² D1-J5 + Novantrone 40 to 60mg/m² D1 (53)	11	53%	-	6 months
Aracytine 1g/m2/12h J1-J5 + Etoposide 100mg/m² J1-J5 + Amsacrine 120 mg/m² J1-3 (47)	40	40%	10%	5.4 months
Fludarabine 30mg/m² D1-J5 + Aracytin 2g D1-J5 + G-CSF (55)	12	83%	-	-
Fludarabine 25mg/m² 5D + Aracytine 2g 5D + IDA 12 mg/m² x3D (51)	22	42%	-	13 weeks
Hyper CVAD (52)	66	44%		42 weeks
Augmented Hyper CVAD (50)	88	47%	44%	6 months
Novantrone 8mg/m² x 3J, + Etoposide 100mg/m² x 5J + Ifosfamide 1.5g /m2 x 5J (54)	11	73%	-	234 days

More recently, the use of Blinatummomab, Nelarabine in the treatment of T-ALL, Inotuzumab Ozogamicin and immonotherapies using modified T lymphocytes called Chimeric Antigen Receptore Modified T Cells (CAR t-cell) (57,58) have improved both the CR rate and OS.

2.1.7 ***Survival study***

2.1.7.1 *Overall survival*

The OS rate was 36% at 5 years. This rate is higher than that reported in the previous local series (7) (12% at 5 years), comparable to that reported by various series in the literature ranging from 30 to 60% (15-17,19,25,44) but remains lower than the result of GRAALL 2005 (22) (table XLVI).

Table XLVI: Study of OS in adult ALL.

Series	Protocol	Number of patients	SG is 5 years old
Our series Sfax	GRAALL 03/05	39	36%
***Nasf* 1999(7) Sfax**	LALA 76, 87 and HPS 89	58	12%
***Thomas* 2004 (16)**	LALA 94	922	33%

France			
Huget **2009 (15)** **France**	GRAALL 2003	225	60% (42 months)
Huguet **2018 (22)** **France**	GRAALL 2005	787	58,5
Annino **2002 (17) Italy**	GIMEMA ALL0288	794	27% (9 years)
Bassan **2009(19) Italy**	NILG-ALL 09/00	236	34%
Larson 1998 **Chicago**	CALGB	198	43%
Hassan **2012 (26)** **Emirates**	UKALLXII/ECOG E2993	99	-
Stock **2013 (34)** **Chicago**	CALGB 19802	163	30%
Kenneth **2016 (38)** **Australia**	LAM Protocol	20	36,8%
Willington **2018 (25)** **Brazil**	GMALL07/2003	59	15.3 (6 years)

2.1.7.1.1 Patient-related prognostic factors for OS:

> **Sex**

Sex does not appear to be a prognostic factor, contrary to what has been reported in paediatric series where male sex is associated with a poor prognosis. In our series, male sex had no influence on OS (36 vs 37%). Only one study showed a greater OS in women (59).

> **Age**

In our series, OS was better for patients aged < 40 years, although the difference was not statistically significant (p= 0.312).

Both remission time and overall survival vary with patient age. Survival decreases progressively with age, reaching survival rates of less than 10% in patients aged over 60 (42).

2.1.7.1.2 Disease-related prognostic factors

> **Initial leukocytosis**

Initial hyperleukocytosis is a poor prognostic factor associated with poorer OS. It was even considered to be the poorest prognostic factor in B-ALL, with an overall survival of 19% to 29% (60,61). In T-line ALL, however, the prognostic value of white blood cells has been recognised for very high values of around 100 G/l. In our series, OS was better for non-hyperleukocytic forms (< 30 G/L) (41%) compared with hyperleukocytic forms (25%), but not significantly so (p=0.492).

> **The phenotype**

Overall survival at 5 years was slightly better for B- than for T-AL (39% vs. 32%) without the difference being significant; these results were also reported in the series published by *Annino* (17). However, for most series in the literature, the T phenotype is correlated with better OS than the B phenotype (18,23,27,34) (Table XLVII).

Table XLVII: Study of OS in adult ALL according to phenotype.

Serie	% SG		P
	LAL B	LAL T	
Our series **Sfax**	39	32	0,925
***Bouallegue* 2011 (23) Sousse**	58,3	83,1	0,02
***Stock* 2013 (34) Chicago**	25	53	0,035
***Kantarjian* 2000 (27) Chicago**	32,6	36,5	0,46
***Larson 1998*(18) Chicago**	39	60	0,05
***Hassan* 2012 (26) Emirates**	49,7	60	-
***Annino* 2002 (17) Italy**	30	27	-

> **The presence of cytogenetic abnormalities**

In our series, OS was better for patients with a normal karyotype than for those with a pathological karyotype, but the difference was not significant (35% vs 21%). This was observed in the Sousse series with a significant difference (49.4 vs 25% with p= 0.05). According to the literature, a complex karyotype, t(4;11) and t(8,14) are correlated with poor OS (31).

2.1.7.1.3 Prognostic factors related to response to treatment

> **Corticosensitivity**

The 5-year OS was better for corticosensitive patients than for corticoresistant patients (38 vs. 25%). The prognostic role of corticosensitivity was demonstrated by the GIMEMA group, showing an 8-year OS of 33% for corticosensitive patients and 17% for corticoresistant patients (P=0.0001) (17).

> **Chemosensitivity**

In our series, chemosensitivity was correlated with better OS, although the difference was not significant (44 vs 20%).

> **The treatment group**

In our series, the OS of high-risk patients was greater than that of standard-risk patients (40 vs 28%). This could be explained by the small number of standard-risk patients and the improved response to allogeneic transplantation.

> **Allografts**

In our series, allogeneic bone marrow transplantation was associated with a better 5-year OS with a significant difference (P=0.013); this finding was also found in various series in the literature (62,63).

2.1.7.2 *Relapse-free survival*

The 5-year SRH in our series was 46%. It was better than that observed in the former local series (12%) (7), comparable to the Sousse series (43.2%) (23) and close to that reported by the various series in the literature, varying from 30 to 59% (15) (Table XLVIII).

Table XLVIII: SSR at 5 years for the different series in the literature.

Series	Protocol	SSR at 5 years old % of SSR at 5 years old
Our series	GRAALL	46

Sfax		
Nasfi 1999 (7) Sfax	LALA76, 87 and HPS 89	12
Bouallegue 2012 (23) Sousse	Hyper CVAD	43.2 (24 months)
Thomas 2004 (16) France	LALA 94	30
Huguet 2009 (15) France	GRAALL 2003	59 (42 months)
Bassan 2009 (19) Emirates	NILG-ALL 09/00	33
Stock 2013 (44) Chicago	CALGB 19802	35
Kenneth 2016 (38) Australia	LAM Protocol	44,1

In our series, chemosensitivity and the absence of a tumour syndrome had a statistically significant influence on SRH (0.05 and 0.028 respectively). These parameters have not been studied in the literature.

Corticosensitivity is correlated with better SSR, both in our series (51 vs 25% p=) and in the *Annino* and *Thomas* series (p= 0.0003 and 0.02 respectively) (16,17).

The risk group did not correlate with better SRH in our series. However, in the series published by *Huguet* (15), SRH was better for patients treated in the STD group than in the RE group, with a statistically significant difference (68 vs 52%, p=0.05).

Allograft significantly improves SSR, both in our series and in the series published by *Thomas* (45 vs 23% p=0.007) (16).

2.1.7.3 *Event-free survival*

The 5-year SES in our series was 39%. It was better than that observed in the previous local series (12%) (7) (due to fewer induction deaths) but lower than that reported by the GRAALL 2003 and 2005 studies (Table XLIX).

Table XLIX: SES at 5 years for different series in the literature.

Series	Protocol	SES at 5 years (%)
Our series Sfax	GRAALL Tunisian	39
Nasf 1999 (7) Sfax	LALA 76, 87 and HPS 89	12
Bouallegue 2011 (23) Sousse	Hyper CVAD	47.3 (24 months)
Huguet 2009(15) France	GRAALL 2003	55 (42 months)
Huguet 2018 (22) France	GRAALL 2005	52,5
Hassan 2012(26) Emirates	UKALLXII/ECOG E2993	27.8 (3 years)

2.1.7.3.1 Patient-related prognostic factors

> <u>Age</u>

In our series, the SES of patients aged < 40 years was better than that of patients aged > 40 years, although the difference was not significant. According to the literature, an age < 45 years is correlated with a better SES (15,26).

> **Sex**

There was no difference in SES between male and female patients (36 vs 35%). However, male patients had a better SES in the Sousse, *Xu* and *Hassan* series (23,26,64).

2.1.7.3.2 Disease-related prognostic factors

> **Hyperleukocytosis**

In our series, non-hyperleukocytic forms (<30 G/L) were associated with a better SES (39 vs 20%). This was comparable with the Sousse series (23).

> **The phenotype**

In our series, phenotype B ALL correlated with a better SES without the difference being significant (38 vs 32%). In the Sousse series and the various series in the literature, phenotype T had a better SES than phenotype B (23,26,65).

> **Cytogenetic abnormalities**

In our series, the 5-year SES was 34% for patients with a normal karyotype and 20% for those with a pathological karyotype (p= 0.757). In the Sousse series the SES was better for normal karyotypes with a significant difference (74.1 vs 50%, p= 0.05) (23).

2.1.7.3.3 Prognostic factors related to response to treatment

> **Corticosensitivity**

The SES of our corticosensitive patients is better than that of corticoresistant patients (36 vs 25%) without the difference being significant. This has also been demonstrated by *Cortes* (37).

> **Chemosensitivity**

In our series, chemosensitivity improved SES without the difference being statistically significant (48 vs 20). In the study published by *Cortes*, chemoresistance was correlated with poor SES with a significant p of 0.00006 (37).

> **The risk group**

In our series, there was no difference in terms of patient SES.
treated according to the STD group compared with those treated according to the RE group.

This could be explained by the improved SES of the RE group after allografting.

> **Allogeneic bone marrow transplants**

Allogeneic bone marrow transplantation statistically significantly improved SES both in our series and in the series published by *Rowe* (66).

2.2 LAL phi+ :

The phi+ chromosome is the result of a reciprocal translocation between chromosomes 9 and 22, resulting in a fusion of the BCR (breakpoint cluster region) gene on chromosome 22 with the ABL (abelson tyrosine kinase) gene on chromosome 9. This t(9;22) (q34;q11) encodes a BCR-ABL protein with tyrosine kinase activity.

2.2.1 *Study of complete remission*

The overall CR rate in our series was 90% (70% after one treatment and a gain of 20%

after the 2eme treatment). This rate is comparable to different series in the literature ranging from 93 to 97% (67-73) (Table L).

Table L: Rates of CR, relapse and induction death in phi+ ALL from different series in the literature.

Series	Protocol	Deces induction (%)	RC (%)	Relapse (%)
Our Tunisia series	GRAAPH Tunisien 2005	10	90	33
***Labarthe* 2006 (72) France**	GRAAPH 2003	6	96	18
***Chalandon* 2015 (71) France**	GRAAPH 2005	3,7	94,8	-
***Lee* 2005 (73) Korea**	Imatinib + intensive chemotherapy	5	95	31
***Wassmann* 2006 (69) Germany**	GMALL 06/99 and 07/03	-	95	-
Thomas 2010 (70) Texas	Hyper CVAD + Imatinib	-	93	24
***Wang* 2017 (67) China**	CODP (induction), hyper CVAD (consolidation)	2,1	95,8	22
***Hatta* 2017(68) Japan**	ALL202 (Imatinib 600 mg)	3	97	38

2.2.2 *Fall*

In our series, 33% of our phi+ ALL patients had an isolated medullary relapse during follow-up. This rate is comparable to different series in the literature where the relapse rate varied between 18 and 38% (70,73,74) (Table L).

2.2.3 *Study of deaths*

In our series, the rate of death during induction treatment was 10% higher than that reported in the literature (2.1 to 5%) (67,68,7173) (Table L).

2.2.4 *Survival study*

2.2.4.1 *Overall survival*

The 5-year OS in our series was 50%, comparable to different series in the literature ranging from 43 to 69% (67-73) (Table LI).

Table LI: SG of phi+ LALs from different series in the literature.

Series	Protocol	SG(%)
Our Tunisia series	GRAAPH Tunisien 2005	50
***Labarthe* 2006 (72) France**	GRAAPH 2003	65 (18 months)
***Chalandon* 2015 (71) France**	GRAAPH 2005	45,6
***Lee* 2005(73) Korea**	Imatinib + intensive chemotherapy	60 (26 months)
***Wassmann* 2006 (69) Germany**	GMALL 06/99 and 07/03	43 (2 years)
***Thomas* 2010 (70) Texas**	Hyper CVAD + Imatinib	54 (3 years)
***Hatta* 2017(68) China**	ALL202 (Imatinib 600 mg)	50 (5 years)

***Wang* 2017 (67) Japan**	CODP (induction), hyper CVAD (consolidation)	69.2 (4 years)

Age, sex and the presence of a tumour syndrome do not influence OS either in our series or in the literature (67,68). However, a WBC count < 30000 elt/mm^3 is correlated with OS in our series and in the literature (67,68,75).

Allogeneic bone marrow transplantation significantly improves OS in various series in the literature (67,68,71,75,76), and this was also observed in our series (Table LII).

Table LII: OS of phi+ ALL from different series in the literature according to allograft.

Series	SG (%)	P
Our Tunisia series	80 vs. 20	0,145
Chalandon 2015 (71) France	-	0,002
***Hatta* 2017(68) China**	-	< 0,001
***Bassan* 2010 (75) Italy**	50 vs 16	0,00
***Seol* 2017 (76) Korea**	-	0,000
***Wang* 2017(67) Japan**	82.6 vs 46.5	< 0,001

2.2.4.2 *Relapse-free survival*

The SSR in our series was 58% at 12 months, comparable to the different series in the literature which vary between 43 and 60.9% (67,68,72) (Table LIII).

Table LIII: SSR of phi+ ALL from different series in the literature.

Series	SSR % OF
Our Tunisia series	58 (12 months)
***Hatta* 2017(68) China**	43 (5 years)
***Labarthe* 2006 (72) France**	51 (18 months)
***Wang* 2017 (67) Japan**	60.9 (4years)

In our series, SRH was better for patients aged under 40 (50 vs 25%) and for allograft patients (80 vs 33%), although the difference was not statistically significant. The WBC rate had no influence on SRH (53 vs 66%).

In the various series in the literature, an age < 40 years and a WBC level < 30 G/L are correlated with a better SSR (67,74). Allogeneic transplantation is associated with a better RFS both in our series and in the literature (Table LIV).

Table LIV: SSR of phi+ ALL according to allograft in different series in the literature.

Series	Protocol	Allograft vs non-allograft SSR (%)	P
Our Tunisia series	GRAAPH 2005	80 vs 33	0,116
***Hatta* 2017 (68) China**	ALL202 (Imatinib 600mg)	-	< 0,001
***Chalandon* 2015 (71) France**	GRAAPH 2005	-	0,036
***Wang* 2017 (67) Japan**	CODP (induction), hyper CVAD (consolidation)	71.3 vs 43.9	< 0,001

2.2.4.3 ***Event-free survival***

In our series, the SES at 5 years was 40%, comparable to the various series in the literature (table LV).

Table LV: SES of phi+ LALs from different literature series.

Series	Protocol	SES (%)
Our Tunisia series	GRAAPH 2005	40
***Chalandon* (71) France**	GRAAPH 2005	37,1
***Fielding* (77) London**	UKALLXII/ECOG2993	33

An age > 40 years is correlated with poor SES both in our series and in different series in the literature (71). Male sex (33 vs 42) and WBC levels had no influence on SES. Allogeneic transplantation improved EES but the difference was not significant (75 vs 20). This could be explained by the small size of our population.

3 The role of MRD in assessing response

3.1 Definition :

At the time of diagnosis, the tumour mass is estimated to be at least 10^{12} leukemic cells. The classic definition of complete remission is the presence of less than 5% blasts on the myelogram. However, the residual tumour mass not detected by cytological analysis may be as high as 10^{10} cells - this is residual disease.

The current aim of improved therapy is to achieve complete remission with a low level of DRM.

3.2 Resources :

Evaluation of MRD is possible by PCR detection of the fusion transcript or clonal rearrangement of immunoglobulin and T receptor (TCR) genes, or by flow cytometry detection of an aberrant phenotype expressed by blasts at diagnosis (78).

3.2.1 ***Flow cytometry:***

It involves the detection of an aberrant phenotype expressed by blast cells and not expressed by normal hematopoietic cells (79). CF is a rapid, simple and less expensive method than the molecular biology technique (80), but the reliability of the results depends on the number and especially the quality (sensitivity and stability) of the markers tested and also the number of colours used. A better sensitivity and specificity was observed with the use of 4 or more colours (80). The sensitivity threshold of CF for the evaluation of MRD is 10^{-3} to 10^{-4} (79).

322 ***Molecular biology (PCR) :***

It consists of amplifying either a molecular marker of clonality represented by the rearrangement of immunoglobulin or T receptor (TCR) genes, or a fusion transcript specific to the blast cell.

The PCR technique has a sensitivity ranging from 10-4 to 10-6 cells (79).

3.2.3 ***Results and therapeutic benefits:***

Whatever the method used, the level of MRD is classified as :

Low level: MRD $<10^{-4}$: low risk of relapse.

-High level: MRD >10-4: high risk of relapse.

The presence of detectable MRD at a threshold greater than 10^{-4} after induction is strongly predictive of relapse (5,80,81) and consequently poor survival.

In some protocols, even high-risk patients with a negative MRD are considered to have a relatively good prognosis and are no longer candidates for a first-line allograft (5).

Assessment of DRM at several levels during the course of treatment makes it possible to monitor the progress of the disease and detect any relapses in good time, even if they are sub-clinical.

4 Place of hematopoietic growth factors

The use of hematopoietic growth factors (HGF) reduces the incidence and duration of febrile episodes associated with neutropenia (5,33), as well as severe infections. As a result, the induction death rate is reduced, especially in elderly subjects (18).

In addition, the use of FCH appears to be associated with better rates of complete remission in some studies (18).

The advantage of using these FCHs is particularly obvious for high-risk leukaemias, but less so for standard-risk acute lymphoblastic leukaemias (82,83).

5 Neuro-meningeal prophylaxis :

CNS prophylaxis is essential in the treatment of adult ALL, since 30% of CR patients present a neuromeningeal relapse in the absence of this prophylaxis, compared with only 5% with prophylaxis (84).

This prophylaxis is based on a combination of 3 approaches (5,6):

- Use of high doses of intravenous meningeal chemotherapy: MTX HD, Aracytine HD, L-Asparaginase, Dexamethasone.
- Lumbar punctures with intrathecal injection of chemotherapy: MTX + Corticoids + Aracytin.
- Cerebromeningeal irradiation.

In the GRAALL 2005 protocol, this consisted of the administration of 7 LPs (one single LP during the prephase and 6 triple LPs) combined with CNS irradiation. This prophylactic irradiation took place between the end of delayed intensification and the start of maintenance treatment. It includes two lateral fields covering the skull, the base of the skull and the first two cervical vertebrae. Doses are 18 Gy over 10 sessions (5 sessions per week for 2 weeks).

6 Treatment of phi+ ALL with TKIs in combination with chemotherapy:

Imatinib, a 1ere generation TKI, binds to the inactive fragment of the bcr- abl kinase, partially blocking its ATP binding site. This prevents conformational change of the active tyrosine kinase (85).

Dasatinib, a 2eme generation inhibitor, has a more potent inhibition of BCR-ABL kinase activity, being able to bind either the active or inactive form of the ABL kinase domain. It also inhibits SRC family proteins and crosses the meningeal barrier (86).

Nilotinib, a 2eme generation inhibitor, has greater affinity and selectivity for the BCR-ABL kinase than Imatinib, and inhibits the activity of the ABL gene tyrosine kinase and ABL mutants except T 315 I (87).

Ponatinib, a 3eme generation inhibitor, is a potent pan-inhibitor of BCR-ABL with high binding affinity to both native and mutant forms of ABL kinase. It inhibits the tyrosine kinase activity of both the ABL gene and the ABL T315I mutant (88).

The combination of Imatinib with chemotherapy is not associated with an increase in toxicity (5), but rather with an increase in the CR rate, an improvement in overall survival and an increase in the number of patients receiving a CR1 allograft. The CR rate of patients included in the GRAAPH 2003 protocol who benefited from Imatinib was 96%, and the four-year OS rate was 52% for patients treated with Imatinib in combination with alleviated chemotherapy versus 20% before the introduction of TKIs (89). This rate was 54% at three years for patients included in the HCVAD protocol in combination with Imatinib, compared with only 15% for patients receiving the same protocol without Imatinib (62,71).

Dasatinib was initially prescribed for patients resistant or intolerant to Imatinib with satisfactory results: in a study in which 78% of patients had kinase domain mutations (including 20% with the T315 I mutation) a major molecular response and a complete cytogenetic response were obtained in 42% and 58% of cases respectively (86).

In the GIMAMA LAL1205 study, induction combining Dasatinib with corticotherapies for patients with phi+ ALL was associated with a rapid and profound response. At 20 months follow-up, overall survival was 69% and disease-free survival was 51% (90).

More recently, a trial combining Dasatinib with HCVAD-type chemotherapy in 35 patients with previously untreated phi+ ALL showed encouraging results, with a complete remission rate of 94% and a 2-year survival rate of 64% (91).

The use of Nilotinib in phi+ ALL has recently been tested. A published study combining Nilotinib with chemotherapy in patients not initially treated showed: a 4.5 molecular response rate in 91% of cases and a relapse-free survival rate at 2 years in 72% of cases (92).

In the PACE phase II study, 32 phi+ ALL patients were treated with Ponatinib. All were resistant to at least 2 TKIs and 13 patients were resistant to at least three TKIs: a major hematological response was obtained in 41% of cases, a major cytogenetic response in 47% and a complete cytogenetic response in 38% of cases (88).

In our series, all patients were initially treated with chemotherapy in combination with Imatinib according to a protocol inspired by the GRAAPH 2005 protocol. Three patients were resistant to Imatinib, two of whom were treated in 2eme line with Dasatinib. The 3eme patient did not receive treatment with a 2eme generation TKI due to unavailability of the treatment.

7 Place of autograft

Autotransplantation uses marrow harvested in remission, possibly treated in vitro with chemotherapy or monoclonal antibodies, in order to eliminate residual disease in the

graft. This marrow is then transfused as for allogenic transplants, after conditioning. Autotransplantation was compared at first remission with post-induction treatments for non-phi+ ALL and no significant difference was demonstrated, although there appeared to be fewer relapses beyond 3 years with autotransplantation (16,93,94).
In addition, autotransplantation continues to have a place in phi+ ALL with no HLA-compatible donors and complete molecular response after 2 courses of chemotherapy. In the GRAAPH 2005 protocol, 29 patients underwent autotransplantation. OS and RFS were comparable between allograft and autograft patients (71).

8 Place of allograft

Allogeneic bone marrow transplantation is a potentially curative treatment for ALL, especially when used as consolidation therapy in patients with CR1. Its benefits are based on the immunological effect of the graft against leukaemia and, more secondarily, on the dose-intensive effect of conditioning in terms of blast eradication (5).
Given the good results obtained with chemotherapy alone in the STD groups and the high MRT rate, it is only indicated for high-risk patients in order to improve survival (5,33).
After a relapse, allograft transplantation is the best therapeutic alternative in CR2 with an OS of 33% compared with 8% for CR2 patients treated with chemotherapy alone (95).
In our series, 13 patients were allografted in CR1: 9 non-phi+ ALL and 4 phi+ ALL. Nine patients are alive in CR, including 6 non-phi+ ALL and 3 phi+ ALL.
The prospective study, LALA87, demonstrated a significant advantage for high-risk patients in terms of SRH of allograft versus chemotherapy alone or in combination with autograft (39 vs 15%). This was also validated in the LALA 94 study, where allograft showed its superiority in terms of SRH for high-risk patients (45 vs 23%) with a significant difference (p=0.007). The beneficial effect of allograft on SES was demonstrated by the *City of Hope and Standfor University* series, with a 5-year SES of 64% and a relapse rate of 15% (96).
In recent years, prognostic stratification based on the level of MRD has made it possible to select a group of very high-risk patients with a positive MRD. These patients alone will be candidates for bone marrow allogeneic transplantation. This criterion has been adapted by the GRAALL 2014 trial, the results of which are currently being published (41).
Because of the seriousness of the phi+ form, most authors recommend intensifying therapy for patients in CR. However, the question that currently arises is whether the initial use of a 2eme generation TKI in combination with chemotherapy will obviate the need for transplantation.
Although the use of chemotherapy in combination with TKIs in the treatment of phi+ ALL increases CR rates to 90%, the majority of patients relapse within 6 to 11 months of starting treatment, justifying intensification by allograft. In fact, 3 studies have demonstrated the benefits of allograft therapy in the treatment of phi+ ALL:

In the JALSG ALL202 study, the risk of relapse was estimated at 13% in the allograft group and 90% in non-allograft patients. Overall survival of allograft patients at 3 years was 65% (74).
The use of Imatinib in combination with hyper CVAD followed by allograft improved overall survival at 3 years by 90% compared with only 33% without allograft(70).
The results of the GRAAPH 2003 protocol combining Imatinib with chemotherapy showed an overall survival at 4 years of 55% with allograft compared with only 25% without allograft (89).
To answer the question of whether it is necessary to combine chemotherapy with TKIs and whether allogeneic bone marrow transplantation is mandatory for patients with complete molecular response in CR1, a clinical trial was launched by the Estern Cooperative Oncology Group/American college of Radiology Imaging Network (ECOG/ACRIN) which randomised Blinatumumab, TKIs and corticosteroids versus TKIs plus chemotherapy. A 2eme randomisation of MRD negative patients between bone marrow allograft and TKI maintenance therapy. The results of this trial have not yet been published.

> ***<u>Use of post-transplant TKIs :</u>***

Is it necessary to prescribe a TKI post allograft? and which TKI should be prescribed? The risk of post allograft relapse is greater if the Bcr-Abl transcript is detectable pre allograft. Some teams recommend treatment with TKIs post allograft to reduce the risk of relapse. A group of experts from the Acute Leukemia Working Party has published recommendations for the use of TKIs post allograft, given the inconclusive results of retrospective studies and the absence of prospective studies. These recommendations include (97):

- Molecular monitoring by testing for the Bcr-abl transcript and determining mutation status should be carried out before and after allogeneic transplantation.
- Monitoring of MRD should begin 4 weeks after allogeneic transplantation. During the 1ere year of treatment, molecular monitoring should be carried out every 6 to 8 weeks on a marrow sample and every 4 to 6 weeks on a peripheral blood sample.
- Patients with undetectable MRD after allogeneic transplantation may receive prophylactic treatment or be monitored until MRD becomes positive.
- Patients who test positive for MRD after allogeneic transplantation should receive prophylactic treatment with TKIs as soon as possible.
- ^{ere}The 1st-line treatment is Imatinib at a dose of 400 mg/d. Patients with early molecular relapse (within 3 months post allograft) or BCR-ABL levels greater than 10^{-4} at any time post allograft should be treated with 2eme generation TKIs (Nilotinib 200 mg/d or Dasatinib 50-100 mg/d). The 2eme generation TKIs should be used in the event of resistance to Imatinib or if there is a kinase domain mutation either pre or post allograft. A switch to a 2eme generation TKI is recommended if the Bcr-Abl transcript is detectable 6 to 8 weeks after transplantation.
- Patients with central nervous system disease should be treated with Dasatinib.
- TKI treatment should be continued for 12 months following MRD negativation for

allograft patients in CR1. For those who have been allografted into CR2 or late remission, treatment should be prescribed for life unless there are problems of tolerance or safety. Individual adjustments may be necessary in cases of severe toxicity.

- Undesirable hematological and extra-hematological effects must be monitored according to the toxicity of each type of TKI.

9 Adolescent and young adult ALL (AYA) :

The definition of 'AYA' varies between research teams. Some define it as patients aged between 15 and 18 years, while others define it as patients aged over 25 years (40). Compared with children, this group of patients is characterised by a higher frequency of poor prognosis cytogenetic abnormalities and a lower frequency of good prognosis abnormalities (40).

Current therapeutic recommendations for the AYA group favour treatment according to protocols inspired by paediatric protocols. The therapeutic results are very encouraging:

-Survival rates ranged from 67% to 78% for AYA treated with paediatric protocols, compared with 34% to 41% for AYA treated with adult protocols.

-The largest prospective study conducted by the US intergroup study (318 AYA treated between 2007 and 2012) showed a toxic DC rate of 3%, OS and SES at 2 years of 79% and 66% (98,99).

The following table reports the therapeutic results of ALL in the AYA group treated with adult versus paediatric protocols in some retrospective studies:

Table LVI: Therapeutic results of AYA according to study group.

Studies/comparison		Number	Age group (years)	Median age (years)	CR rate	Survival rate
United States (100)	CALGB (adult)	124	16-20	19	90%	SG is 7 years old 46
	CCG (paediatric)	197	16-20	16	90%	67%
France (101)	LALA-94(adult)	100	15-20	18	83%	SSE at 5 years 41
	FRALLE-93 (paediatric)	77	15-20	16	94%	67%
Netherlands (102)	HOVON (adult)	73	15-20	20	91%	SSE 5 years old 38
	DCOG (paediatric)	47	15-20	12	98%	71%
United Kingdom (103)	UKLLXII/E2993 (adult)	67	15-17	-	94%	SG at 5 years 56
	ALL97 (paediatric)	61	15-17	-	98%	71%
Finland (104)	Finnish Leukemia (adult)	97	17-25	19	97%	SG is 5 years old 60%.
	NOPHO (paediatric)	128	10-16	13	96%	67%

Our team has included AYA up to 25 years in the child protocol since 2000, and given the encouraging results reported in the work of *Frikha. I* (105), our centre decided to extend the EROTC 58951 child protocol to cover AYA up to 30 years of age in 2009.

10 New therapies :

Recently, new therapeutic agents have been tested in the treatment of adult-onset ALL, with the aim of improving therapeutic results both in the first-line setting and in relapsed or refractory forms.

Several new molecules are currently being developed for the treatment of phi+ ALL: INNO-406, Busutinib, XL228, FTY720, AP24534, DCC2036, PHA-739358 and Sorafenib....

INNO-406 and Bosutinib are SCR and ABL inhibitors. Available orally, they have shown activity against Imatinib-resistant BCR-ABL mutants (106,107).

10.1.1 *Rituximab*

Rituximab is a chimeric anti-CD20 antibody marketed under the brand name Mabthera.

Rituximab is intended for use in CD 20+ B-ALL. Combining this antibody with chemotherapy increases OS and DFS.

The GRAALL 2005 protocol tested the addition of Rituximab to chemotherapy (16 to 18 injections), in 105 patients aged between 15 and 59 years. The 2-year SES in the Rituximab arm was 65% compared with 52% in the no Rituximab arm, with a significant difference (p= 0.04) and no increase in toxicity (108). Rituximab was combined with the HCVAD protocol by the MD Anderson group, resulting, for patients aged under 60 years, in an increase in the duration of CR (70% versus 38% p<0.001), an improvement in overall survival (75% versus 47%) and a reduction in the relapse rate (109). Similar results were obtained in the German group studying adult ALL (110).

10.1.2 *Blinatumommab*

Blinatumommab is a bi-specific antibody: on the one hand it binds selectively to CD19, present in the majority of B-ALL, and on the other hand to CD3 present in the cytotoxic T cell. This binding activates the endogenous T lymphocytes responsible for tumour irradiation. Blinatummomab has been used in both non-phi+ and phi+ ALL. Its prescription for patients with refractory or relapsed non-phi+ ALL has resulted in a CR rate of around 43% (57,111).

Blinatumommab has shown very good results in phi+ ALL: a phase II study testing Blinatumomab in 21 patients (5 phi+ ALL) with positive MRD showed MRD negativation in 80% of cases. After a median follow-up of 33 months, relapse-free survival was 63% (112). A more recent phase II study tested the efficacy of Blinatumomab in 45 patients with resistant and/or relapsed phi+ ALL who had received at least one 2eme generation TKI or who had received Imatinib and were intolerant of the 2eme generation TKI, 36% of patients were in complete remission, including 14 with undetectable MRD (113).

10.1.3 *Inotuzumab ozogamicin*

Inotuzomab ozogamicin (INO) is an anti-CD22 antibody conjugated to calicheamicin. The use of this antibody in the treatment of refractory or relapsed forms of the disease,

in a phase III study involving 218 patients, showed the superiority of the use of INO compared with chemotherapy alone, with 81% CR versus 29% and a higher percentage of negative MRD (78% versus 28% p<0.001)(114).
The use of INO in the treatment of first-line ALL in combination with reduced chemotherapy of the mini HCVAD type in elderly patients has produced encouraging results, with a 98% CR rate, negative MRD in 76%, progression-free survival at 2 years of 52% and overall survival of 66% (114,115).

10.1.4 ***CAR-T cells***

CAR-T cells are T lymphocytes, usually autologous, genetically modified to express a surface receptor capable of directly recognising a specific tumour antigen, the CD19 of blasts (116).
A study published by *M.Davila* (117) in 16 adult patients with refractory ALL B showed a CR rate of 88% with MRD negativity in 75% of cases and a median OS of 9 months. An update of these data on 44 patients confirmed these results, with 84% CR and 83% MRD negative.

11 LAL in the elderly

The definition of older patients differs from team to team. Some teams define older patients on the basis of the possibility of receiving intensive chemotherapy, including stem cell transplantation, generally limited to an age of 55-65 years (118).
In our centre, we opted for a limit of 55 years to define the group of elderly subjects.
The prevalence of ALL in the elderly is 16-31% of all adult ALL. Among the poor prognostic factors in this age group is a high performance status with intolerance to chemotherapy (119). With standard chemotherapy, the mortality rate during induction treatment for subjects aged >60 years is estimated at 42% (118,120). The median survival is 15 months and only 20% of patients are alive after 3 years. Reducing chemotherapy doses while preserving efficacy could improve outcomes in elderly patients with ALL. A prospective study was conducted by the GMALL team involving 268 elderly subjects followed for ALL and treated according to the BFM protocol. The early mortality rate was 14%, of which 6% was in CR. The 5-year CR and OS rates were 78% and 23% respectively (121). In a phase 2 trial of 52 elderly subjects (median age 68 years) treated with INO in combination with mini-HCVD chemotherapy, progression-free survival at 2 years was 59% (115).
In the prospective EWALL PH01 study, 71 elderly subjects with phi+ ALL (median age 69 years) were treated with combination chemotherapy and Dasatinib. The CR rate after induction was 96%. A 3-log reduction in the Bcr-abl ratio after consolidation was observed in 65% of patients. OS at 5 years was 36% (122).
An alternative for phi+ ALL is the use of TKIs as monotherapy in patients whose general condition does not allow chemotherapy to be administered. Imatinib alone or in combination with corticotherapy induces CR rates of the order of 90 to 100% (85).
The 1er prospective randomised trial comparing the therapeutic results of a series of 55 elderly subjects (median age= 68 years) on lmatinib alone versus chemotherapy was published by *Ottmann* in 2007. The CR rate was 96.3% in the Imatinib alone arm

versus 50% in the chemotherapy arm. This high rate is explained by the absence of toxic deaths in the Imatinib arm compared with the standard chemotherapy arm (0% versus 14.8%) (123).

The use of Imatinib alone as monotherapy has certainly led to an improvement in quality of life, but these responses are transient and relapses are very frequent, mainly due to mutations in the kinase domain.

A phase II study tested Nilotinib (at a dose of 400mg/d) in patients resistant or intolerant to Imatinib or refractory phi+ ALL, showing a complete molecular response in 28% of cases, one of whom had negative residual disease (87).

In our series, only one patient, aged 53, was treated with TKI monotherapy after having received 2 courses of chemotherapy due to significant infectious toxicity: she received Imatinib at a dose of 800 mg/d, switched to TKI 2eme generation at 11 months of treatment for an increase in the Bcr-abl ratio and is alive with a good molecular response.

12 Proposals and outlook

> **Non-phi+ ALL**

In our series, we used protocols inspired by the French GRAALL 2003 and 2005 protocols. Our results were better than the previous local series, with notably better CR rates, fewer relapses and toxic deaths, and better survival. The results of our work are encouraging, but remain inferior to those reported by the GRAALL 2005 study, especially in terms of SES (39 vs 52.5%). This could be explained by the high relapse rate in our series (50 vs 29.8%) in both the STD and RE groups.

Improving our results will certainly involve not only improving supportive care, with the aim of improving the death rate in induction and consolidation, but also improving the quality of remission, with the aim of reducing the relapse rate. Intensification of induction chemotherapy, the introduction of Mabthera for CD20+ B-ALL and assessment of residual disease at the end of the course appear to be the essential parameters for intervention.

To improve support processing, we propose..:

1) To treat our patients with ALL in a single room.
2) To install an air filtration system: positive pressure.
3) Better compliance with hygiene conditions.
4) Improved availability of anti-infection and anti-fungal treatments.
5) Improve the quality of labile blood products: transfusion with UPCs and leukocyte-depleted RBCs.

For chemotherapy modifications we propose:

1) To extend the inclusion of our patients up to the age of 60, while adapting chemotherapy doses from the age of 50.
2) To include residual disease in the evaluation of response to treatment and to introduce it into risk group stratification. To do this, in addition to the old criteria:

- For the standard group we require a level of MRD $<10^{-2}$ after the induction cure and a MRD $<10^{-3}$ after the 3eme block.

■ For the high risk group we require an MRD level > 10^{-2} after induction and/or > 10^{-3} after the 3[eme] block.

■ To treat both standard and high risk groups using the same therapeutic regimen. The indication for allogeneic bone marrow transplantation in RC1 still remains for the RE group aged under 50.

3) For the induction cure we offer:

■ Increase the dose of DNR from 45 mg/m^2 /d J8-9; J15-16 to 50mg/m^2 /d J8, J9, J10 and 30mg/m^2 /d J22-23 for subjects aged 30 to 50 years. This dose is reduced to 30mg/m^2 /d D8, D9, D10, D22, D23 for subjects aged 51 to 60.

■ Increase the dose of Endoxan from 500 m^2 /d D8 and D15 to 750 mg/ m^2 /d D8 and D22.

■ To reduce the duration of corticosteroid exposure for subjects aged over 50 from 23 days to 15 days (D1-J15).

4) Blocks B1, B2, B3, B4, B5, B6: same doses.

5) Replace the reinduction and reconsolidation cure with a single cure called delayed intensification (see proposal).

6) Blocks B7, B8, B9: same doses.

7) Radiotherapy of the encephalon: same dose.

8) Maintenance treatment: same doses.

9) Introduction of Mabthera at a dose of 375 mg/m^2 /injection (16 to 18 injections) for CD20+ B-ALL divided as follows:

■ Two injections during the induction treatment: D8 and D15.

■ Two injections during the catch-up treatment: D1 and D7.

■ One injection during the consolidation cure 1 and 3.

■ Two injections during delayed intensification: D1 and D7.

■ One injection during the consolidation cure 7 and 9.

■ One injection during reinduction cycles 1, 3, 5, 7, 9 and 11.

Proposal for a new chemotherapy protocol.

Induction		
Dexamethasone	6 mg/m²	D1 - D14 then D21 to D28 **D1-J15 if age > 50 years**
Vincristine	1.5 mg/m²	D8 - D15 - D22 - D29
Daunorubicin	50 mg/m² in 4H PIV 30 mg/m² in 4H PIV **if > 50 years old, 30 mg/m2 in 4H IVP**	J8, J9, J10 J15,J16 **J8, J9, J10, J15, J16**
PL	triple	D1, D8 and D15, D22
L-Asparaginase	6000U1/m²	J11,J14, J17,J20, J23, J26
Endoxan	750 mg/m² in 1H PIV	D8 and D15
Mabthera	375 mg/m /d²	J8, J15
G-CSF		from D17

Assessment after induction :

A post-induction myelogram should be carried out when the patient emerges from aplasia after this course of treatment, although a 48-hour delay should be observed

between the last injection of G-CSF and the myelogram.
-Control karyotype.
-Assessment of residual disease (MRD1).

Post-induction treatment		
B1: BLOCK ARA-C (blocks 1 and 4) Before each block: CBC: WBC> 2000, PNN> 500, Pq> 100 000, ALAT<5 x Nle, creat clearance > 60 ml/mn		
Aracytin	2g/m² morning and evening IV (3h)	J1 and J2
Dexamethasone	10mg/12h	J1 and J2
L-Asparaginase	10,000 IU/m²	J3
Mabthera	375 mg/m /d²	J1
G-CSF	1fl/J SC	J7a J13
B2 : METHO BLOCK (blocks 2 and 5)		
Vincristine	2 mg total dose	J1
Methotrexate	3 g/ m²	D1 with folinic acid rescue
L-Asparaginase	10,000 IU/m²	IV to J3
Purinethol	60 mg/m²	J1 to J7
G-CSF	1fl/J SC	J8a J13
PL	triple	J2
B3 : Endoxan BLOCK (blocks 3 and 6)		
Cyclophosphamide	500mg/ m², IV (3 h)	J1 and J2
Etoposide (VP16)	75 mg/m²	J1 and J2
Methotrexate	25 mg/m²	J1
Mabthera	375 mg/m /d²	J1
G-CSF	1fl/d SC	J13 up to PNN>1000/ m³
PL	triple	J2
Assessment of residual disease (MRD2).		
Delayed intensification: Begins 7 days after discharge from aplasia in the 6ᵉᵐᵉ block *With PNN>1000/mm³ and Pq>100 000/mm³, ALT <2.5 x Nle, creat clearance > 60 ml/mn		
Dexamethasone	6mg/m²	J1-14 **D1-J7, if age > 50 years**
DNR	30 mg/m² in 4H PIV	J1, J2, J3, 15, 16 **D1, D2, D3 if age > 50 years**
Endoxan	750mg/m²	J1, 15
L-Asparaginase	6000 IU/m²	J8, 10, 12, 10, 20, 22
PL	triple	J 1, J8
GCSF	1fl/d SC	Day 18 until PNN>1000/ m³
Blocks B7 - B8 - B9 15 days apart		
Radiotherapy of the encephalon: at a dose of 18 Gy up to C2 under purinethol without MTX, CBC checked once a week.		
Maintenance treatment: To be started 3 to 4 weeks after B9 block if PNN>1000/mm³ and Pq>100 000/mm³ It lasts for 2 years.		
Purinethol	60 mg/m² per os	Every day
Methotrexate	25 mg/m² / week per os	Every day
PL	**triple**	Every 2 months

Monthly reinduction, for the first year only.		
Oncovin	1.5 mg/m² /day IV (max 2mg/injection)	J1
Prednisone	40 mg/m /d²	J1, J7
If HLA compatible and age < 50 years: Three blocks B1 - B2 - B3 then allograft - If CNS+, radiotherapy from encephalon to C2 - One to 2 stand-by courses of MTX-Aspa may be administered 15 days apart: MTX: 1.5 g/m² D1 infused over 3 hours Asparaginase: 10,000 U/m² D2		

> **LAL phi+.**

In view of the good results obtained by the use of TKIs in combination with reduced chemotherapy in the treatment of adult phi+ ALL, we propose to include adolescents and adults from the age of 20 in the adult protocol (inspired by GRAAPH 2005) (Appendix 3). For patients between 56 and 70 years of age, we propose the EWALL protocol (122), which is dedicated to older subjects and includes an even lighter chemotherapy regimen combined with a TKI, Dasatinib.

Bone marrow allotransplantation certainly retains its place as a first-line treatment, but for patients with a major molecular response after 3eme consolidation and no HLA-compatible donors, we propose HSC autotransplantation as a consolidation treatment.

Proposed treatment for phi+ ALL aged 55 to 70.

Induction		
Dexamethasone	40 mg/m² /d, IV	J1-J2, J8-J9, J15-J16, J22-J23
Oncovin	1 mg	D1, D8, D15 and D22
Dasatinib	140 mg PO (in 1 dose)	D1 to D1 of consolidation
PL triple	Methotrexate 15 mg, Aracytine 40 mg, dexa 4 mg	D9, D16 and D23
Neupogen	^{5}Hg/kg^j	From day 15 to PN >1000/mm3.
Assessment after induction treatment : An informative post-induction myelogram should be carried out on D29 of this first course of treatment, with a 48-hour delay between the last injection of Neupogen and this myelogram, whatever the platelet level. -Control karyotype. Evaluation of residual post-induction BCR-ABL disease must be carried out at this time, on the marrow, before beginning the consolidation treatment (if BCR-M type transcript).		
Consolidation treatment (6 cycles of 4 weeks): Dasatinib 100mg/d from D14 to D27 of each cycle.		
Cure 1/3/5		
Methotrexate	1000 mg/m² as a 3-hour infusion	J1, rescue with folinic acid
Asparaginase	10 000 mg/m²	J2
Triple PL	Methotrexate 15 mg, Aracytine 40 mg, prednisone 40 mg	Cycle 1 and 3
G-CSF	^{5}Hg/ kg^j	If PNN <1000/mm³
Cure 2/4/6		
Aracytin	1 g/ m² /12h in PIV over 2h	J1, J3, J5
G-CSF	Vig/kg/l	If PNN <1000/mm³

Before each consolidation cycle: quantitative BCR-ABL
Maintenance: 7 cycles, 1 cycle every 2 months during the 1ere year and every 3 months during the 2eme year.
Dasatinib 100 mg/d PO, daily for 1 month every 2 months. Purinethol 60 mg/m² /d when Dasatinib is stopped Methotrexate 25 mg/m² /d when Dasatinib is stopped Dexamethasone 40 mg/d D1, D2 (months 8, 10, 12, 15, 18, 21, 24). Vincristine 1 mg IV (months 8, 10, 12, 15, 18, 21, 24).

5 Conclusion

ALL is the leading type of childhood cancer (25% of paediatric cancers) and is the most common of all AL cancers. However, after the age of 15, their intrinsic frequency decreases, as does their proportion within AMLs (< 1% of adult cancers, with 20% of AMLs versus 80% of AMLs). The disease therefore has a bimodal distribution, with an initial peak in children aged between 2 and 5 years and a second peak in adults around the age of 50.

Current treatment of adult ALL is based on intensive chemotherapy inspired by paediatric protocols, leading to improved therapeutic results with a CR rate in excess of 80%, but survival is still unsatisfactory due to a relatively high relapse rate.

Over the last 20 years, several therapeutic alternatives have been used to improve outcomes, including allogeneic bone marrow transplantation, the use of chemotherapy inspired by paediatric protocols and, above all, the use of TKIs in combination with chemotherapy in the treatment of phi+ ALL.

The aim of this retrospective study was to evaluate the therapeutic outcomes, prognostic factors and survival of 49 adult patients with ALL treated according to GRAALL- and GRAAPH-inspired protocols between January 2004 and December 2015.

For this purpose, we designed a form collecting epidemiological, diagnostic, therapeutic and evolutionary data. The statistical methods used were the Chi2 (X2) test for correlation, the Kaplan-Meier method for survival, and the Logrank test and Cox model for comparisons.

There were 49 patients, 23 males and 26 females, with a sex ratio of 0.88. The median age was 42 years, with extremes ranging from 20 to 56 years. The median age was 42 years, with extremes ranging from 20 to 56 years. 55% of our patients were over 40 years of age.

At the time of diagnosis, anemic syndrome was noted in 84% of cases, haemorrhagic syndrome in 26%, infectious syndrome in 32% and tumour syndrome in 63%. No testicular involvement was noted. 5% of our patients had CNS involvement.

The median white blood cell count was 10 G/L. Leukocytosis of less than 30 G/L was noted in 72% of cases, in 16% of cases the WBC count was between 30 G/L and 100 G/L and hyper leukocytosis >100 G/L in 12% of cases.

The median hemoglobin level was 7.5 g/dL with extremes from 2.4 g/dL to 14.6 g/dL. A hemoglobin level < 10 g/dL was found in 73% of cases.

Thrombocytopenia was observed in 43 patients, and was less than 50 G/L in 59% of cases.

B-ALL occurred in 65% of cases, T-ALL in 33% and biphenotypic acute leukaemia (B + myeloid) in 2%.

BCR-ABL rearrangement and/or t(9,22) were found in 22% of our patients.

The cytogenetic study was conclusive in only 33 patients, 49% of whom had a normal karyotype. Cytogenetic abnormalities were noted in 51% of cases. The t (9,22) was found in 6 cases.

Forty-six of our ALL patients received protocol treatment: 36 non-phi+ patients and 10 patients (appendix 6).

For the group of non-phi+ ALL patients:

Corticosensitivity was found in 89% of cases and the only predictive factor was a WBC level <10 G/l.

Chemosensitivity at day 15 was noted in 84% of cases and the only predictive factor was corticoresensitivity.

Seven patients died during the induction treatment (19%), including 4 before therapeutic evaluation. Thirty patients had CR after 2 courses of chemotherapy, giving an overall CR rate of 93% (90% after one course). The therapeutic failure rate was estimated at 5%.

Seven patients were treated in the STD group (20%) and twenty-three in the RE group (80%). Among the 28 patients in CR who continued their treatment, 20 patients were indicated for OM allografting in CR1: 9 were transplanted, 6 of these patients were VV in CR and 3 were DCD (2 toxic DC and one post allograft relapse).

Of the 19 non-allograft patients, 6 were VV in CR (including 2 STD and 4 RE) and 13 were DCD (1 maintenance toxic death and 12 due to disease progression).

During our study we noted 14 relapses (50%): 3 cases belonging to the STD group, among the 6 who continued their treatment (i.e. 50%) and 11 to the RE group (50%). The median time to relapse was 9 months compared with CR of (20 and 6 months in the STD and RE groups respectively). Allogeneic bone marrow transplantation was the only factor influencing the occurrence of relapse.

With a median follow-up of 92 months, OS was 39% at 5 years. The only influencing factor was allogeneic bone marrow transplantation in CR1.

SRH was 47% at 5 years. The absence of a tumour syndrome, chemosensitivity at D15 and allogeneic bone marrow transplantation were predictive of a better follow-up rate.

SES was 39% at 5 years. Allogeneic bone marrow transplantation was the only influencing factor.

For the group of phi+ ALL patients:

Only one patient died during the induction treatment (10%).

The overall CR rate was 90% (after induction 70% with a gain of 20% after catch-up).

Of the 9 patients in CR, 8 were indicated for OM allograft in CR1 and only 4 were transplanted: 3 patients were VV in CR and 1 patient was DCD due to GVH iiiguK.

Of the 5 non-allograft patients: 2 are VV (one in CR1 and one in CR2) and 3 are DCD (1 toxic death and 2 deaths due to progression of the disease).

In our series we noted 3 relapses (33% of cases).

For a median follow-up of 57 months, the OS, RSG and SES at 5 years were 50, 58 and 40% respectively.

❖ It's true that our results are better than in the past, but a lot of work remains to be done to improve these results even further:

- Improving hospital conditions and support treatments to further reduce the rate of toxic deaths.

- Respecting the block deadlines to insist on the principle of intensive dose chemotherapy recommended in the therapeutic protocols. This involves increasing the department's inpatient capacity to compensate for delays in treatment.
- To obtain the Bcr Abl transcript result rapidly, before D8, in order to diagnose phi+ ALL in time for treatment with reduced chemotherapy in combination with TKIs.
- To carry out HLA typing quickly, so that our patients can be allografted in good time before a relapse occurs.
- Start bone marrow autotransplantation at our centre in order to intensify treatment for phi+ donor-negative ALL.

With this new proposal for stratifying patients into risk groups, assessing response based on residual disease and the new therapeutic protocol, we hope to achieve better results, which will soon be evaluated in prospective studies.

Bibliography

1. **Baranger L, Cuccuini W, Lefebvre C, Luquet I, Perot C, Radford I, et al.** Cytogenetics in the management of children and adult acute lymphoblastic leukemia (ALL): an update by the Groupe francophone de cytogenetique hematologique (GFCH). Ann Biol Clin (Paris). 20169-10;(5):547-560.
2. **Boissel N.** Therapeutiques cibleses dans les leucemies aig^s. Reanimation. 2006 Aug;15(4):278-84.
3. **Bray F, Ferlay J, Laversanne M, Brewster DH, Gombe Mbalawa C, Kohler B, et al.** Cancer Incidence in Five Continents: Inclusion criteria, highlights from Volume X and the global status of cancer registration: Cancer Incidence in Five Continents Volume X. Int J Cancer. 2015 Nov 1;137(9):2060-71.
4. **Huguet F, Recher C**. Acute leukemia in adults. Hematologie. 2011 5-6;(3):203-224.
5. **L. Farnault, J. Boudjarane, V. Baccini, R. Costello.** Acute lymphoblastic leukaemia in adults. Hematology. 2015; S1155-1984(14)62406-7
6. **Paul S, Kantarjian H, Jabbour EJ**. Adult Acute Lymphoblastic Leukemia. Mayo Clin Proc. 2016 Nov;91(11):1645-66.
7. **Nasfi S**. Les leucemies aigues lymphoblastiques de l'adulte: aspects diagnostiques, therapeutiques et evolutifs (a propos de 58 observation).These de medecine; 1999. TH/SF1269
8. **Hdiji S**. Prise en charge des LAL en Tunisie, etude multicentrique, Societe Tunisienne d'Hematologie 2008.
9. **Thomas X, Pavan L, Le Q-H.** Adult acute lymphoblastic leukemia with central nervous system involvement: an update. Bull Cancer (Paris). 2008 Jul 1;95(7):707-15.
10. **Florence binder F et al.** national estimate of the incidence of malignant hemopathies.2013
11. **Jabbour EJ, Faderl S, Kantarjian HM.** Adult Acute Lymphoblastic Leukemia. Mayo Clin Proc. 2005 Nov;80(11):1517-27.
12. **Bassan R, Gatta G, Tondini C, Willemze R.** Adult acute lymphoblastic leukaemia. Crit Rev Oncol Hematol. 2004 Jun;50(3):223-61.
13. **Hourigan M, Goldstone A. Anjali A S, Lazarus H M, et al.** Adult Acute Lymphocytic Leukemia: biology and treatment. New York: Springer; 2011. :77- 87.
14. **Gargouri M.** Etudes epidemiologiques et cytologiques des leucemies aigues en hematologie a Sfax: a propos de 531 cas. Memoire de fin d'etudes pharmaceutiques. Monastir; 2003.
15. **Huguet F, Leguay T, Raffoux E, Thomas X, Beldjord K, Delabesse E, et al.** Pediatric-Inspired Therapy in Adults With Philadelphia Chromosome-Negative Acute Lymphoblastic Leukemia: The GRAALL-2003 Study. J Clin Oncol. 2009 Feb 20;27(6):911-8.
16. **Thomas X, Boiron J-M, Huguet F, Dombret H, Bradstock K, Vey N, et al.** Outcome of Treatment in Adults With Acute Lymphoblastic Leukemia: Analysis of the LALA-94 Trial. J Clin Oncol. 2004 Oct 15;22(20):4075-86.

17. **Annino L, Maria Luce V, Andrea C, Giorgina S, et al.** Treatment-of-adult-acute-lymphoblastic-leukemia-ALL-long-term-follow-up-of-the-GIMEMA-ALL-0288-randomized-study. Blood. 2002 Feb 1; 99 (3):863-71.
18. **Larson RA, Dodge RK, Linker CA, Stone RM, Powell BL, Lee EJ, et al.** A randomized controlled trial of filgrastim during remission induction and consolidation chemotherapy for adults with acute lymphoblastic leukemia: CALGB study 9111. Blood. 1998 Sep 1;92(5):1556-64.
19. **Bassan R, Spinelli O, Oldani E, Intermesoli T, Tosi M, Peruta B, et al.** Improved risk classification for risk-specific therapy based on the molecular study of minimal residual disease (MRD) in adult acute lymphoblastic leukemia (ALL). Blood. 2009 Apr 30;113(18):4153-62.
20. **Gokbuget N, Arnold R, Bohme A, Fietkau R, Freund M, Ganser A, et al.** Improved Outcome in High Risk and Very High Risk ALL by Risk Adapted SCT and in Standard Risk ALL by Intensive Chemotherapy in 713 Adult ALL Patients Treated According to the Prospective GMALL Study 07/2003. Blood. 2007 Nov 16;110(11):12.
21. **Ribera J-M, Oriol A, Bethencourt C, Parody R, Hernandez-Rivas J-M, Moreno M-J, et al.** Comparison of intensive chemotherapy, allogeneic or autologous stem cell transplantation as post-remission treatment for adult patients with high-risk acute lymphoblastic leukemia. Results of the PETHEMA ALL-93 trial. Haematologica. 2005 Oct;90(10):1346-56.
22. **Huguet F, Chevret S, Leguay T, Thomas X, Boissel N, Escoffre-Barbe M, et al.** Intensified Therapy of Acute Lymphoblastic Leukemia in Adults: Report of the Randomized GRAALL-2005 Clinical Trial. J Clin Oncol. 2018 Aug 20;36(24):2514-23.
23. **Bouallegue S**. Treatment of acute lymphoblastic leukemia in adults using the hyper CVAD protocol in 30 cases. These de medecine de Mounastir;TH/MO2292.
24. **Ben Neji.H, Jaber.D, Ahour.M, Ben Abdennebi.Y, Aissaoui.L**. Adult-onset acute lymphoblastic leukemia : feasibility of the protocol GRALL2005.Societe Tunisienne d'Hematologie. 2013.
25. **Fernandes da Silva Junior W, Medina AB, Yamakawa PE, Buccheri V, Velloso EDRP, Rocha V.** Treating Adult Acute Lymphoblastic Leukemia in Brazil-Increased Early Mortality Using a German Multicenter Acute Lymphoblastic Leukemia-based regimen. Clin Lymphoma Myeloma 2018 Mar;
26. **Hassan IB, Kristensen J, Alizadeh H, Bernsen R.** Outcome of patients with acute lymphoblastic leukemia (ALL) following induction therapy with a modified (pulsed dexamethasone rather than continuous prednisone) UKALL XII/ECOG E2993 protocol at Tawam Hospital, United Arab Emirates (UAE). Med Oncol. 2013 Jun;30(2).
27. **Kantarjian HM, O'Brien S, Smith TL, Cortes J, Giles FJ, Beran M, et al.** Results of Treatment With Hyper-CVAD, a Dose-Intensive Regimen, in Adult Acute Lymphocytic Leukemia. J Clin Oncol. 2000 Feb;18(3):547-547.

28. **Arber DA, Orazi A, Hasserjian R, Thiele J, Borowitz MJ, Le Beau MM, et al.** The 2016 revision to the World Health Organization classification of myeloid neoplasms and acute leukemia. Blood. 2016 May 19;127(20):2391-405.
29. **Group Fran^ais de Cytogenetique Hematologique.** Cytogenetic abnormalities in adult acute lymphoblastic leukemia: correlations with hematologic findings outcome. Blood. 1996 Apr 15;87(8):3135-42.
30. **Charrin C.** A report from the LALA-94 and LALA-SA groups on hypodiploidy with 30 to 39 chromosomes and near-triploidy: 2 possible expressions of a sole entity conferring poor prognosis in adult acute lymphoblastic leukemia (ALL). Blood. 2004 Jun 29;104(8):2444-51.
31. **Moorman AV, Harrison CJ, Buck GAN, Richards SM, Secker-Walker LM, Martineau M, et al.** Karyotype is an independent prognostic factor in adult acute lymphoblastic leukemia (ALL): analysis of cytogenetic data from patients treated on the Medical Research Council (MRC) UKALLXII/Eastern Cooperative Oncology Group (ECOG) 2993 trial. Blood. 2007 Apr 15;109(8):3189-97.
32. **Lara D, Gauthier M.** Acute lymphocytic leukemia. Hematology. 2014 3-4;(2):116-129.
33. **Acute lymphoblastic leukaemia of adults**. Hematology. 2010 Sep;(spec3):15-19.
34. **Stock W, Johnson JL, Stone RM, Kolitz JE, Powell BL, Wetzler M, et al.** Dose intensification of daunorubicin and cytarabine during treatment of adult acute lymphoblastic leukemia: Results of Cancer and Leukemia Group B Study 19802. Cancer. 2013 Jan 1;119(1):90-8.
35. **Inoue C, Sobue S, Aoyama Y, Mizutani N, Kawamoto Y, Nishizawa Y, et al.** BCL2 inhibitor ABT-199 and JNK inhibitor SP600125 exhibit synergistic cytotoxicity against imatinib-resistant Ph+ ALL cells. Biochem Biophys Rep. 2018 Sep;15:69-75.
36. **Thomas DA.** Philadelphia Chromosome Positive Acute Lymphocytic Leukemia: A New Era of Challenges. Hematology. 2007 Jan 1;2007(1):435-43.
37. **Cortes J, Fayad L, O'Brien S, Keating M, Kantarjian H.** Persistence of Peripheral Blood and Bone Marrow Blasts during Remission Induction in Adult Acute Lymphoblastic Leukemia Confers a Poor Prognosis Depending on Treatment Intensity. Clin Cancer Res. 1999 Sep 1;5(9):2491.
38. **Bradstock KF, Morley A, Byth K, Szer J, Prosser I, Cannell P, et al.** Effects of intensive induction and consolidation chemotherapy with idarubicin and high dose cytarabine on minimal residual disease levels in newly diagnosed adult precursor- B acute lymphoblastic leukemia. Contemp Clin Trials Commun. 2016 Dec;4:9-13.
39. **Pui C-H, Robison LL, Look AT.** Acute lymphoblastic leukaemia. The Lancet. 2008 Mar;371(9617):1030-43.
40. **Narayanan S, Shami PJ.** Treatment of acute lymphoblastic leukemia in adults. Crit Rev Oncol Hematol. 2012 Jan;81(1):94-102.
41. **Summary of the GRAALL_2014 study protocol**. (synopsis) Version 1.1.
42. **Rowe JM.** Induction therapy for adults with acute lymphoblastic leukemia: results of more than 1500 patients from the international ALL trial: MRC UKALL XII/ECOG

E2993. Blood. 2005 Dec 1;106(12):3760-7.
43. **Cornelissen JJ, van der Holt B, Verhoef GEG, van 't Veer MB, van Oers MHJ, Schouten HC, et al.** Myeloablative allogeneic versus autologous stem cell transplantation in adult patients with acute lymphoblastic leukemia in first remission: a prospective sibling donor versus no-donor comparison. Blood. 2009 Feb 5;113(6):1375-82.
44. **Stock W, Johnson JL, Stone RM, Kolitz JE, Powell BL, Wetzler M, et al.** Dose intensification of daunorubicin and cytarabine during treatment of adult acute lymphoblastic leukemia: Results of Cancer and Leukemia Group B Study 19802. Cancer. 2013 Jan 1;119(1):90-8.
45. **Frey NV, Luger SM.** How I treat adults with relapsed or refractory Philadelphia chromosome-negative acute lymphoblastic leukemia. Blood. 2015 Jul 30;126(5):589.
46. **Oriol A, Vives S, Hernandez-Rivas JM, Tormo M, Heras I, Rivas C, et al.** Outcome after relapse of acute lymphoblastic leukemia in adult patients included in four consecutive risk-adapted trials by the PETHEMA Study Group. Haematologica. 2010 Apr 1;95(4):589-96.
47. **Reman O, Buzyn A, Lheritier V, Huguet F, Kuentz M, Stamatoullas A, et al.** Rescue therapy combining intermediate-dose cytarabine with amsacrine and etoposide in relapsed adult acute lymphoblastic leukemia. Hematol J. 2004;5(2):123-9.
48. **Abbi KKS, Rybka W, Ehmann WC, Claxton DF.** Phase I/II Study of Clofarabine, Etoposide, and Mitoxantrone in Patients With Refractory or Relapsed Acute Leukemia. Clin Lymphoma Myeloma Leuk. 2015 Jan;15(1):41-6.
49. **Aldoss I, Pullarkat V, Patel R, Watkins K, Mohrbacher A, Levine AM, et al.** An effective reinduction regimen for first relapse of adult acute lymphoblastic leukemia. Med Oncol. 2013 Dec;30(4).
50. **Faderl S, Thomas DA, O'Brien S, Ravandi F, Garcia-Manero G, Borthakur G, et al.** Augmented Hyper-CVAD Based on Dose-Intensified Vincristine, Dexamethasone, and Asparaginase in Adult Acute Lymphoblastic Leukemia Salvage Therapy. Clin Lymphoma Myeloma Leuk. 2011 Feb;11(1):54-9.
51. **Yavuz S, Paydas S, Disel U, Sahin B.** IDA-FLAG Regimen for the Therapy of Primary Refractory and Relapse Acute Leukemia: A Single-Center Experience: Am J Ther. 2006 Sep;13(5):389-93.
52. **Koller CA, Kantarjian HM, Thomas D, O'Brien S, Rios MB, Kornblau S, et al.** The hyper-CVAD regimen improves outcome in relapsed acute lymphoblastic leukemia. Leukemia. 1997 Dec;11(12):2039-44.
53. **Raanani P, Shpilberg O, Gillis S, Avigdor A, Hardan I, Berkowicz M, et al.** Salvage therapy of refractory and relapsed acute leukemia with high dose mitoxantrone and high dose cytarabine. Leuk Res. 1999 Aug;23(8):695-700.
54. **Schiller G, Lee M, Territo M, Gajewski J, Nimer S.** Phase II study of etoposide, ifosfamide, and mitoxantrone for the treatment of resistant adult acute lymphoblastic leukemia. Am J Hematol. 1993 Jul;43(3):195-9.
55. **Montillo M, Tedeschi A, Centurioni R, Leoni P.** Treatment of Relapsed Adult

Acute Lymphoblastic Leukemia with Fludarabine and Cytosine Arabinoside Followed by Granulocyte Colony-Stimulating Factor (FLAG-GCSF). Leuk Lymphoma. 1997 Jan;25(5-6):579-83.
56. **Camera A, Annino L, Chiurazzi F, Fazi P, Cascavilla N, Fabbiano F, et al.** GIMEMA ALL - Rescue 97: a salvage strategy for primary refractory or relapsed adult acute lymphoblastic leukemia. Haematologica. 2004 Feb;89(2):145-53.
57. **Topp MS, Gokbuget N, Stein AS, Zugmaier G, O'Brien S, Bargou RC, et al.** Safety and activity of blinatumomab for adult patients with relapsed or refractory B-precursor acute lymphoblastic leukaemia: a multicentre, single-arm, phase 2 study. Lancet Oncol. 2015 Jan;16(1):57-66.
58. **Gokbuget N, Basara N, Baurmann H, Beck J, Bruggemann M, Diedrich H, et al.** High single-drug activity of nelarabine in relapsed T-lymphoblastic leukemia/lymphoma offers curative option with subsequent stem cell transplantation. Blood. 2011 Sep 29;118(13):3504-11.
59. **Durrant IJ, Grant Prentice H, Richards SM.** Intensification of treatment for adults with acute lymphoblastic leukaemia: results of U.K. Medical Research Council randomized trial UKALL XA. Br J Haematol. 1997 Oct;99(1):84-92.
60. **Xavier Thomas, Hussam Saad, Denis Fiere.** Prognosis and treatment of acute lymphoblastic leukaemia in adults. Hematology. 2000.
61. **Faderl S, O'Brien S, Pui C-H, Stock W, Wetzler M, Hoelzer D, et al.** Adult acute lymphoblastic leukemia: Concepts and strategies. Cancer. 2010 Mar 1;116(5):1165-76.
62. **Pidala J, Djulbegovic B, Anasetti C, Kharfan-Dabaja M, Kumar A.** Allogeneic hematopoietic cell transplantation for adult acute lymphoblastic leukemia (ALL) in first complete remission. Cochrane Haematological Malignancies Group, editor. Cochrane Database Syst Rev. 2011 Oct 5
63. **Yanada M, Matsuo K, Suzuki T, Naoe T.** Allogeneic hematopoietic stem cell transplantation as part of postremission therapy improves survival for adult patients with high-risk acute lymphoblastic leukemia: A metaanalysis. Cancer. 2006 Jun 15;106(12):2657-63.
64. **Xu W, Li J-Y, Qian S-X, Wu H-X, Lu H, Chen L-J, et al.** Outcome of treatment with Hyper-CVAD regimen in Chinese patients with acute lymphocytic leukemia. Leuk Res. 2008 Jun;32(6):930-5.
65. **Kang W, Hahn JS, Kim JS, Cheong J-W, Yang WI.** Nine-Year Survival of Lymphoblastic Lymphoma Patients. Yonsei Med J. 2006;47(4):466.
66. **Rowe J, Richards S, Burnett A, Wiernik P, Harrison G, Lazarus H, et al.** Favorable results of allogeneic bone marrow transplantation (BMT) for adults with Philadelphia (Ph)-chromosome-negative acute lymphoblastic leukemia (ALL) in first complete remission (CR): Results from the International ALL trial (MRC UKALL XII/ECOG E2993). BLOOD. 2001;98(11):481A-481A.
67. **Wang J, Jiang Q, Xu L, Zhang X-H, Chen H, Qin Y-Z, et al.** Allogeneic Stem Cell Transplantation versus Tyrosine Kinase Inhibitors Combined with Chemotherapy

in Patients with Philadelphia Chromosome-Positive Acute Lymphoblastic Leukemia. Biol Blood Marrow Transplant. 2018 Apr;24(4):741- 50.

68. **Hatta Y, Mizuta S, Matsuo K, Ohtake S, Iwanaga M, Sugiura I, et al.** Final analysis of the JALSG Ph+ALL202 study: tyrosine kinase inhibitor-combined chemotherapy for Ph+ALL. Ann Hematol [Internet]. 2018 Apr 24 [cited 2018 Aug 5]; Available from: http://link.springer.com/10.1007/s00277-018-3323-8

69. **Wassmann B.** Alternating versus concurrent schedules of imatinib and chemotherapy as front-line therapy for Philadelphia-positive acute lymphoblastic leukemia (Ph+ALL). Blood. 2006 May 9;108(5):1469-77.

70. **Thomas DA, O'Brien SM, Faderl S, Ravandi Kashani F, Wierda WG, Andreeff M, et al.** Long-term outcome after hyper-CVAD and imatinib (IM) for de novo or minimally treated Philadelphia chromosome-positive acute lymphoblastic leukemia (Ph-ALL). J Clin Oncol. 2010 May 20;28(15_suppl):6506-6506.

71. **Chalandon Y, Thomas X, Hayette S, Cayuela J-M, Abbal C, Huguet F, et al.** Randomized study of reduced-intensity chemotherapy combined with imatinib in adults with Ph-positive acute lymphoblastic leukemia. Blood. 2015 Jun 11;125(24):3711-9.

72. **de Labarthe A, Rousselot P, Huguet-Rigal F, Delabesse E, Witz F, Maury S, et al.** Imatinib combined with induction or consolidation chemotherapy in patients with de novo Philadelphia chromosome-positive acute lymphoblastic leukemia: results of the GRAAPH-2003 study. Blood. 2007 Feb 15;109(4):1408-13.

73. **Lee K-H, Lee J-H, Choi S-J, Lee J-H, Seol M, Lee Y-S, et al.** Clinical effect of imatinib added to intensive combination chemotherapy for newly diagnosed Philadelphia chromosome-positive acute lymphoblastic leukemia. Leukemia. 2005 Sep;19(9):1509-16.

74. **Hatta Y, Mizuta S, Ohtake S, Sugiura I, Ueda Y, Kanamori H, et al.** Promising Outcome of Imatinib-Combined Chemotherapy Followed by Allogeneic Hematopoietic Stem Cell Transplantation for Philadelphia Chromosome-Positive Acute Lymphoblastic Leukemia: Results of the Japan Adult Leukemia Study Group (JALSG) Ph+ALL202 Regimen. Blood. 2009 Nov 20;114(22):3090.

75. **Bassan R, Rossi G, Pogliani EM, Di Bona E, Angelucci E, Cavattoni I, et al.** Chemotherapy-Phased Imatinib Pulses Improve Long-Term Outcome of Adult Patients With Philadelphia Chromosome-Positive Acute Lymphoblastic Leukemia: Northern Italy Leukemia Group Protocol 09/00. J Clin Oncol. 2010 Aug;28(22):3644-52.

76. **Seol CA, Cho Y-U, Jang S, Park C-J, Lee J-H, Lee J-H, et al.** Prognostic significance of recurrent additional chromosomal abnormalities in adult patients with Philadelphia chromosome-positive acute lymphoblastic leukemia. Cancer Genet. 2017 Oct;216-217:29-36.

77. **Fielding AK, Rowe JM, Buck G, Foroni L, Gerrard G, Litzow MR, et al.** UKALLXII/ECOG2993: addition of imatinib to a standard treatment regimen enhances long-term outcomes in Philadelphia positive acute lymphoblastic leukemia.

Blood. 2014 Feb 6;123(6):843-50.
78. **Berry DA, Zhou S, Higley H, Mukundan L, Fu S, Reaman GH, et al.** Association of Minimal Residual Disease With Clinical Outcome in Pediatric and Adult Acute Lymphoblastic Leukemia: A Meta-analysis. JAMA Oncol. 2017 Jul 13;3(7):e170580.
79. **van Dongen JJM, van der Velden VHJ, Bruggemann M, Orfao A.** Minimal residual disease diagnostics in acute lymphoblastic leukemia: need for sensitive, fast, and standardized technologies. Blood. 2015 Jun 25;125(26):3996-4009.
80. **Campana D.** Minimal Residual Disease in Acute Lymphoblastic Leukemia. Hematology. 2010 Dec 1;2010(1):7-12.
81. **Monika Bru'ggemann, Thorsten Raff, Thomas Flohr, Nicola Go "kbuget, Makoto Nakao, Jo Droese, et al.** Clinical significance of minimal residual disease quantification in adult patients with standard-risk acute lymphoblastic leukemia. neoplasia. 2005 Sep 29;
82. **Ottmann O, Hoelzer D, Gracien E, Ganser A, Kelly K, Reutzel R, et al.** Concomitant granulocyte colony-stimulating factor and induction chemoradiotherapy in adult acute lymphoblastic leukemia: a randomized phase III trial. Blood. 1995 Jul 15;86(2):444.
83. **Geissler K, Koller E, Hubmann E, Niederwieser D, Hinterberger W, Geissler D, et al.** Granulocyte colony-stimulating factor as an adjunct to induction chemotherapy for adult acute lymphoblastic leukemia--a randomized phase-III study. Blood. 1997 Jul 15;90(2):590-6.
84. **Jabbour E, Thomas D, Cortes J, Kantarjian HM, O'Brien S.** Central nervous system prophylaxis in adults with acute lymphoblastic leukemia: current and emerging therapies. Cancer. 2010 May 15;116(10):2290-300.
85. **Ravandi F, Kebriaei P.** Philadelphia Chromosome-Positive Acute Lymphoblastic Leukemia. Hematol Oncol Clin North Am. 2009 Oct;23(5):1043-63.
86. **Ottmann O, Dombret H, Martinelli G, Simonsson B, Guilhot F, Larson RA, et al.** Dasatinib induces rapid hematologic and cytogenetic responses in adult patients with Philadelphia chromosome positive acute lymphoblastic leukemia with resistance or intolerance to imatinib: interim results of a phase 2 study. Blood. 2007 Oct 1;110(7):2309-15.
87. **Ottmann OG, Larson RA, Kantarjian HM, le Coutre PD, Baccarani M, Hochhaus A, et al.** Phase II study of nilotinib in patients with relapsed or refractory Philadelphia chromosome-positive acute lymphoblastic leukemia. Leukemia. 2013 Jun;27(6):1411-3.
88. **Cortes JE, Kim D-W, Pinilla-Ibarz J, le Coutre P, Paquette R, Chuah C, et al.** A Phase 2 Trial of Ponatinib in Philadelphia Chromosome-Positive Leukemias. N Engl J Med. 2013 Nov 7;369(19): 1783-96.
89. **Tanguy-Schmidt A, Rousselot P, Chalandon Y, Cayuela J-M, Hayette S, Vekemans M-C, et al.** Long-Term Follow-Up of the Imatinib GRAAPH-2003 Study in Newly Diagnosed Patients with De Novo Philadelphia ChromosomePositive Acute

Lymphoblastic Leukemia: A GRAALL Study. Biol Blood Marrow Transplant. 2013 Jan;19(1):150-5.

90. **Foa R, Vitale A, Vignetti M, Meloni G, Guarini A, De Propris MS, et al.** Dasatinib as first-line treatment for adult patients with Philadelphia chromosomepositive acute lymphoblastic leukemia. Blood. 2011 Dec 15;118(25):6521-8.

91. **Benjamini O, Dumlao TL, Kantarjian H, O'Brien S, Garcia-Manero G, Faderl S, et al.** Phase II trial of HyperCVAD and Dasatinib in patients with relapsed Philadelphia chromosome positive acute lymphoblastic leukemia or blast phase chronic myeloid leukemia. Am J Hematol. 2014 Mar;89(3):282-7.

92. **Kim D-Y, Joo Y-D, Lim S-N, Kim S-D, Lee J-H, Lee J-H, et al.** Nilotinib combined with multiagent chemotherapy for newly diagnosed Philadelphiapositive acute lymphoblastic leukemia. Blood. 2015 Aug 6;126(6):746-56.

93. **Marks DI.** Treating the "Older" Adult With Acute Lymphoblastic Leukemia. Hematology. 2010 Dec 1;2010(1):13-20.

94. **Popat U, Carrum G, Heslop HE.** Haemopoietic stem cell transplantation for acute lymphoblastic leukaemia. Cancer Treat Rev. 2003 Feb;29(1):3-10.

95. **Tavernier E, Boiron J-M, Huguet F, Bradstock K, Vey N, et al.** Outcome of treatment after first relapse in adults with acute lymphoblastic leukemia initially treated by the LALA-94 trial. Leukemia. 2007 Sep;21(9):1907-14.

96. **Jamieson CHM, Amylon MD, Wong RM, Blume KG.** Allogeneic hematopoietic cell transplantation for patients with high-risk acute lymphoblastic leukemia in first or second complete remission using fractionated total-body irradiation and high- dose etoposide: a 15-year experience. Exp Hematol. 2003 Oct;31(10):981-6.

97. **Giebel S, Czyz A, Ottmann O, Baron F, Brissot E, Ciceri F, et al.** Use of tyrosine kinase inhibitors to prevent relapse after allogeneic hematopoietic stem cell transplantation for patients with Philadelphia chromosome-positive acute lymphoblastic leukemia: A position statement of the Acute Leukemia Working Party of the: TKIs After AlloHSCT in Ph+ ALL. Cancer. 2016 Oct;122(19):2941- 51.

98. **Curran E, Stock W.** How I treat acute lymphoblastic leukemia in older adolescents and young adults. Blood. 2015;125(24):3702-3710. Blood. 2015 Oct 8;126(15):1868-1868.

99. **Stock W et al.** Early Results from the Phase II C10403 Trial of Combination Chemotherapy for Older Adolescents and Young Adults with Newly Diagnosed ALL ASH 2014, abstract 796.

100. **Stock W, La M, Sanford B, Bloomfield CD, Vardiman JW, Gaynon P, et al.** What determines the outcomes for adolescents and young adults with acute lymphoblastic leukemia treated on cooperative group protocols? A comparison of Children's Cancer Group and Cancer and Leukemia Group B studies. Blood. 2008 Sep 1;112(5):1646-54.

101. **Boissel N, Auclerc M-F, Lheritier V, Perel Y, Thomas X, Leblanc T, et al.**

Should Adolescents With Acute Lymphoblastic Leukemia Be Treated as Old Children or Young Adults? Comparison of the French FRALLE-93 and LALA-94 Trials. J Clin Oncol. 2003 Mar;21(5):774-80.

102. **de Bont JM, van der Holt B, Dekker AW, van der Does-van den Berg A, Sonneveld P, Pieters R.** Adolescents with acute lymphatic leukaemia achieve significantly better results when treated following Dutch paediatric oncology protocols than with adult protocols. Ned Tijdschr Geneeskd. 2005 Feb 19;149(8):400-6.

103. **Ramanujachar R, Richards S, Hann I, Goldstone A, Mitchell C, Vora A, et al.** Adolescents with acute lymphoblastic leukaemia: Outcome on UK national paediatric (ALL97) and adult (UKALLXII/E2993) trials. Pediatr Blood Cancer. 2007 Mar;48(3):254-61.

104. **Usvasalo A, Raty R, Knuutila S, Vettenranta K, Harila-Saari A, Jantunen E, et al.** Acute lymphoblastic leukemia in adolescents and young adults in Finland. Haematologica. 2008 Aug 1;93(8):1161-8.

105. **Frikha I.** Evaluation du protocole EORTC 58951 modifie dans le traitement des leucemies aigues lymphoblastiques : A propos de 134 cas, These pour obtention de doctorat en medecine, SFAX, 2006.

106. **Kantarjian H, Coutre P le, Cortes J, Pinilla-Ibarz J, Nagler A, Hochhaus A, et al.** Phase 1 study of INNO-406, a dual Abl/Lyn kinase inhibitor, in Philadelphia chromosome-positive leukemias after imatinib resistance or intolerance. Cancer. 2010;NA-NA.

107. **Gambacorti-Passerini C, Kantarjian HM, Kim D-W, Khoury HJ, Turkina AG, Brttmmendorf TH, et al.** Long-term efficacy and safety of bosutinib in patients with advanced leukemia following resistance/intolerance to imatinib and other tyrosine kinase inhibitors: Bosutinib in Patients with Advanced Leukemia. Am J Hematol. 2015 Sep;90(9):755-68.

108. **Maury S, Chevret S, Thomas X, Heim D, Leguay T, Huguet F, et al.** Rituximab in B-Lineage Adult Acute Lymphoblastic Leukemia. N Engl J Med. 2016 Sep 15;375(11):1044-53.

109. **Thomas DA, O'Brien S, Faderl S, Garcia-Manero G, Ferrajoli A, Wierda W, et al.** Chemoimmunotherapy With a Modified Hyper-CVAD and Rituximab Regimen Improves Outcome in De Novo Philadelphia Chromosome-Negative Precursor B-Lineage Acute Lymphoblastic Leukemia. J Clin Oncol. 2010 Aug 20;28(24):3880-9.

110. **Hoelzer D, Huettmann A, Kaul F, Irmer S, Jaekel N, Mohren M, et al.** Immunochemotherapy with Rituximab Improves Molecular CR Rate and Outcome In CD20+ B-Lineage Standard and High Risk Patients; Results of 263 CD20+ Patients Studied Prospectively In GMALL Study 07/2003. Blood. 2010 Nov 19;116(21):170.

111. **Kantarjian H, Stein A, Gokbuget N, Fielding AK, Schuh AC, Ribera J-M, et al.** Blinatumomab versus Chemotherapy for Advanced Acute Lymphoblastic Leukemia. N Engl J Med. 2017 Mar 2;376(9):836-47.

112. **Topp MS, Kufer P, Gokbuget N, Goebeler M, Klinger M, Neumann S, et**

al. Targeted Therapy With the T-Cell-Engaging Antibody Blinatumomab of Chemotherapy-Refractory Minimal Residual Disease in B-Lineage Acute Lymphoblastic Leukemia Patients Results in High Response Rate and Prolonged Leukemia-Free Survival. J Clin Oncol. 2011 Jun 20;29(18):2493-8.

113. **Martinelli G, Boissel N, Chevallier P, Ottmann O, Gokbuget N, Topp MS, et al.** Complete Hematologic and Molecular Response in Adult Patients With Relapsed/Refractory Philadelphia Chromosome-Positive B-Precursor Acute Lymphoblastic Leukemia Following Treatment With Blinatumomab: Results From a Phase II, Single-Arm, Multicenter Study. J Clin Oncol Off J Am Soc Clin Oncol. 2017 Jun 1;35(16):1795-802.

114. **Kantarjian HM, DeAngelo DJ, Stelljes M, Martinelli G, Liedtke M, Stock W, et al.** Inotuzumab Ozogamicin versus Standard Therapy for Acute Lymphoblastic Leukemia. N Engl J Med. 2016 Aug 25;375(8):740-53.

115. **Kantarjian H, Ravandi F, Short NJ, Huang X, Jain N, Sasaki K, et al.** Inotuzumab ozogamicin in combination with low-intensity chemotherapy for older patients with Philadelphia chromosome-negative acute lymphoblastic leukaemia: a single-arm, phase 2 study. Lancet Oncol. 2018 Feb;19(2):240-8.

116. **Androulla MN, Lefkothea PC.** CAR T-cell Therapy: A New Era in Cancer Immunotherapy. Curr Pharm Biotechnol. 2018 May 31;19(1):5-18.

117. **Davila ML, Riviere I, Wang X, Bartido S, Park J, Curran K, et al.** Efficacy and Toxicity Management of 19-28z CAR T Cell Therapy in B Cell Acute Lymphoblastic Leukemia. Sci Transl Med. 2014 Feb 19;6(224):224ra25-224ra25.

118. **Gokbuget N.** How I treat older patients with ALL. Blood. 2013 Aug 22;122(8):1366-75.

119. **Go kbuget N.** Treatment of older patients with acute lymphoblastic leukemia. Hematology. 2016 Dec 1;2016(1):573-9.

120. **O'Brien S, Thomas DA, Ravandi F, Faderl S, Pierce S, Kantarjian H.** Results of the hyperfractionated cyclophosphamide, vincristine, doxorubicin, and dexamethasone regimen in elderly patients with acute lymphocytic leukemia. Cancer. 2008 Oct 15;113(8):2097-101.

121. **Goekbuget N, Beck J, Brueggemann M, Burmeister T, Buss EC, Frickhofen N, et al.** Moderate Intensive Chemotherapy Including CNS-Prophylaxis with Liposomal Cytarabine Is Feasible and effective in Older Patients with Ph-Negative Acute Lymphoblastic Leukemia (ALL): Results of a Prospective Trial From the German Multicenter Study Group for Adult ALL (GMALL). Blood. 2012 Nov 16;120(21):1493.

122. **Rousselot P, Coude MM, Gokbuget N, Gambacorti Passerini C, Hayette S, Cayuela J-M, et al.** Dasatinib and low-intensity chemotherapy in elderly patients with Philadelphia chromosome-positive ALL. Blood. 2016 Aug 11;128(6):774- 82.

123. **Ottmann OG, Wassmann B, Pfeifer H, Giagounidis A, Stelljes M, Dtthrsen U, et al.** Imatinib compared with chemotherapy as front-line treatment of elderly patients with Philadelphia chromosome-positive acute lymphoblastic leukemia (Ph+ALL). Cancer. 2007 May 15;109(10):2068-76.

Appendix 1: GRAALL 2003 protocol.

INDUCTION: common for RS and RE groups		
Dexamethasone	6mg/m2	D1 - D14 then D21 to D28
Vincristine	1.5mg/m2	D8 - D15 - D22 - D29
Daunorubicin	45mg/m2 in 4H IVP	D8, D9 and D15, D16
PL	triple	D1, D8 and D15, D22
L-Asparaginase	6000U1/m²	J11,J14, J17,J20, J23, J26
G-CSF		from D17
Standard risk group		
IB cure: Theoretically starts between D36 - D45, if RC with PNN>1000 /mm3 and Pq>100 000 /mm3		
Cytarabine	75mg/m2	J3-6, 10-13, 17-20, 24-27
6-mercaptopurine	60mg/m2	J1-28
PL triple		J3, 17
Cyclophosphamide	1 g/m²	J1, J28
Mesna	1g/m2/d in 3 injections	J1, J28
Intermediate treatment: Begins 14 days after the end of the IB treatment * If WBC>1500/mm3, PNN>500/mm3 and Pq>50 000/mm3		
6-mercaptopurine	25mg/m²	J1 a 56
Methotrexate	5g/m²	D8, D22, D36, D50
PL	triple	J9, J23, J37, J51
Folinic acid	25 mg/m² per os or IV every 6H/12 injections	
Reinduction II A: Begins 14 days after the end of intermediate treatment *With WBC> a 1500/mm3, PNN>500/mm3 and Pq>50 000/mm3		
Dexamethasone	6mg/m²	J1 to 21
Vincristine	1.5g/m² (max 2mg)	J8, J15, J22, J29
Adriamycin	30mg/m²	J8, J15, J22, J29
L-Asparaginase	6000 IU/m²	D8, D11, D15, D18
Reconsolidation II B		
Cytarabine	75 mg/m² IV bolus	J 38 to 41; J45 to J48
6- mercaptopurine	60mg/m²	J 36-49
PL triple		J 38 and J 49
Cyclophosphamide	1 g/m²	J 36
Mesna	1 g/m² in 3 injections	J 36
Radiotherapy of the encephalon: at a dose of 18 Gy up to C2 (at the start of maintenance treatment) under purinethol without MTX, CBC checked once a week.		
Maintenance treatment: To be started 14 days after the end of protocol II Its duration is 112 weeks (24 months) divided into periods of 70 days (10 weeks).		
Purinethol	50 mg/m² per os	J1 to J70
Methotrexate	20 mg/m² / week per os	J1 to J70
PL	triple	Every 2 months
Oncovin	1.5mg/m² /d IV (max 2mg/injection)	J57 and J63
Dexamethasone	6mg/m² /d IV	J57>J63
High risk group		
B1: BLOCK ARA-C (block 1 and 4) Before each block: CBC: WBC> 2000, PNN> 500, Pq> 100 000, ASAT/ ALAT/BilT + C/Ph Alc, creatinemia		

Aracytin	2g/m^2 morning and evening IV (3h)	J1 and J2
Dexamethasone	10 mg/12h	J1 and J2
L-Asparaginase	10,000 IU/m^2	J3
GCSF	1 fl/J SC	J7a J13
B2 : METHO BLOCK (blocks 2 and 5)		
Vincristine	2 mg total dose	J1
Methotrexate	3 g/ m^2	D1 with folinic acid rescue
L-Asparaginase	10,000 IU/m^2	IV to J3
Purinethol	60 mg/m^2	J1 to J7
GCSF	1fl/J SC	J8a J13
PL	triple	J2
B3 : Endoxan BLOCK (blocks 3 and 6)		
Cyclophosphamide	500 mg/ m2, IV (3 h)	J1 and J2
Etoposide (VP16)	75 mg/m2	J1 and J2
Methotrexate	25 mg/m2	J1
GCSF de	1 fl/J SC	J13 up to PN>1000/ m^3
PL	triple	J2
Reinduction **II A:** Begins 14 days after the end of intermediate treatment *With WBC> a 1500/mm3, PNN>500/mm3 and Pq>50 000/mm^3		
Dexamethasone	6 mg/m2	J1-21
Vincristine	1.5 g/m2 (max 2mg)	J8, 15, 22, 29
Adriamycin	30 mg/m2	J8, 15, 22, 29
L-Asparaginase	6000 IU/m2	J8, 11, 15,18
Reconsolidation II B		
Cytarabine	75 mg/m2 IV bolus	J 38-41; J45 to J48
6- mercaptopurine	60 mg/m2	J 36-49
PL triple		J 38
Cyclophosphamide	1 g/m2	J 36
Mesna	1 g/m2 in 3 injections	J 36
Blocks B1 - B2 - B3 15 days apart		
Radiotherapy of the encephalon: at a dose of 18 Gy up to C2 (at the start of maintenance treatment) under purinethol without MTX, CBC checked once a week.		
Maintenance treatment: To be started 14 days after the end of protocol II Its duration is 112 weeks (24 months) divided into periods of 70 days (10 weeks).		
Purinethol	50 mg/m^2 per os	J1 to J70
Methotrexate	20 mg/m^2 / week per os	J1 to J70
PL	triple	Every 2 months
Oncovin	1.5 mg/m^2 /day IV (max 2mg/injection)	J57 and J63
Dexamethasone	6 mg/m^2 /d IV	J57>J63
After the 6 periods of 70 days (60 weeks), patients will receive only purinethol and methotrexate orally for a total of 112 weeks.		

If HLA-matched donor and age < 40 years: Three blocks B1 - B2 - B3 then allograft

- If CNS+, radiotherapy from encephalon to C2
- One to 2 stand-by courses of MTX-Aspa can be administered 15 days apart:

MTX: 1.5 g/m^2 D1 infused over 3 hours

Asparaginase: 10,000 U/m2 D2

Appendix 2: GRAALL 2005 protocol

Induction: common for RS and RE groups		
Dexamethasone	6 mg/m²	D1 - D14 then D21 to D28
Vincristine	1.5 mg/m²	D8 - D15 - D22 - D29
Daunorubicin	45 mg/m² in 4H PIV	D8, D9 and D15, D16
PL	**triple**	D1, D8 and D15, D22
L-Asparaginase	6000U1/m²	J11,J14,J17,J20,J23, J26
Endoxan	500 mg/m² in 1H PIV	D8 and D15
G-CSF		from D17
If remission fails: remedial treatment		
Idarubicin	12 mg/m²	J1 to J3
Aracytin	2000 mg/m² morning and evening, IV (3h)	from J1a J4
G-CSF	150 pg/m /d²	J9 to granular recovery
Standard risk group		
IB cure: Theoretically starts between D36 - D45 If RC with PNN>1000 /mm3 and Pq>100 000/mm³		
Cytarabine	75 mg/m²	J3-6, 10-13, 17-20, 24-27
6-mercaptopurine	60 mg/m²	J1-28
PL triple		J3, 21
Cyclophosphamid e	1 g/m²	J1, 28
Mesna	1g/m2/d in 3 injections	J1, 28
Intermediate treatment: Begins 14 days after the end of the IB treatment * If WBC>1500/mm³ , PNN>500/mm³ and Pq>50 000/mm³		
6-mercaptopurine	25 mg/m²	J1-56
Methotrexate	5 g/m²	J8, 22, 36, 50
PL	triple	J9, 23, 37, 51
Folinic acid	25 mg/m2 per os or IV every 6H/12 injections	
Reinduction II A: Starts 14 days after fi *With WBC> a n of intermediate treatment 1500/mm³ , PNN>500/mm³ el Pq>50 000/mm³		
Dexamethasone	6 mg/m²	J1-21
Vincristine	1.5 g/m² (max 2mg)	J8, 15, 22, 29
Adriamycin	30 mg/m²	J8, 15, 22, 29
L Asparaginase	6000 IU/m²	J8, 11, 15,18
Reconsolidation II B		
Cytarabine	75 mg/m² IV bolus	J 38-41; J45 to J48
6- mercaptopurine	60 mg/m²	J 36-49
PL	triple	J 38
Cyclophosphamide	1 g/m²	J 36
Mesna	1 g/m² in 3 injections	J 36
Radiotherapy of the encephalon: at a dose of 18 Gy up to C2 (at the start of maintenance treatment) under purinethol without MTX, CBC checked once a week.		
Maintenance treatment: To begin 14 days after the end of protocol II Its duration is 112 weeks (24 months) divided into periods of 70 days (10 weeks).		
Purinethol	50 mg/m² per os	J1 to J70
Methotrexate	20 mg/m² / week per os	J1 to J70
PL	triple	Every 2 months
Oncovin	1.5 mg/m² /day IV (max 2mg/injection)	J57 and J63

Dexamethasone	6 mg/m^2 /d IV	J57>J63
High risk group		
B1: BLOCK ARA-C (block 1 and 4) Before each block: CBC: WBC> 2000, PNN> 500, Pq> 100 000, ASAT/ ALAT/BilT + C/Ph Alc, creatinemia		
Aracytin	2g/m^2 morning and evening IV (3h)	J1 and J2
Dexamethasone	10 mg/12h	J1 and J2
L-Asparaginase	10,000 IU/m^2	J3
GCSF	1 fl/J SC	J7a J13
B2 : METHO BLOCK (blocks 2 and 5)		
Vincristine	2 mg total dose	J1
Methotrexate	3 g/ m^2	D1 with folinic acid rescue
L-Asparaginase	10,000 IU/m^2	IV to J3
Purinethol	60 mg/m^2	J1 to J7
GCSF	1fl/J SC	J8a J13
PL	triple	J2
B3 : Endoxan BLOCK (blocks 3 and 6)		
Cyclophosphamide	500 mg/ m2, IV (3 h)	J1 and J2
Etoposide (VP16)	75 mg/m2	J1 and J2
Methotrexate	25 mg/m2	J1
GCSF de	1 fl/J SC	J13 up to PN>1000/ m^3
PL	triple	J2
Reinduction **II A:** Begins 14 days after the end of intermediate treatment *With WBC> a 1500/mm3, PNN>500/mm3 and Pq>50 000/mm^3		
Dexamethasone	6 mg/m2	J1-21
Vincristine	1.5 g/m2 (max 2mg)	J8, 15, 22, 29
Adriamycin	30 mg/m2	J8, 15, 22, 29
L-Asparaginase	6000 IU/m2	J8, 11, 15,18
Reconsolidation II B		
Cytarabine	75 mg/m2 IV bolus	J 38-41; J45 to J48
6- mercaptopurine	60 mg/m2	J 36-49
PL triple		J 38
Cyclophosphamide	1 g/m2	J 36
Mesna	1 g/m2 in 3 injections	J 36
Blocks B1 - B2 - B3 15 days apart		
Radiotherapy of the encephalon: at a dose of 18 Gy up to C2 (at the start of maintenance treatment) under purinethol without MTX, CBC checked once a week.		
Maintenance treatment: To be started 14 days after the end of protocol II Its duration is 112 weeks (24 months) divided into periods of 70 days (10 weeks).		
Purinethol	50 mg/m^2 per os	J1 to J70
Methotrexate	20 mg/m^2 / week per os	J1 to J70
PL	triple	Every 2 months
Oncovin	1.5 mg/m^2 /day IV (max 2mg/injection)	J57 and J63
Dexamethasone	6 mg/m^2 /d IV	J57>J63
After the 6 periods of 70 days (60 weeks), patients will receive only purinethol and methotrexate orally for a total of 112 weeks.		

If HLA-matched donor and age < 50 years: Three blocks B1 - B2 - B3 then allograft

- If CNS+, radiotherapy from encephalon to C2
- One to 2 stand-by courses of MTX-Aspa can be administered 15 days apart:

MTX: 1.5 g/m² D1 infused over 3 hours

Asparaginase: 10,000 U/m2 D2

Appendix 3: GRAAPH 2005 protocol

Induction

Dexamethasone	6 mg/m² /d in 2 injections, IV	D1 - D14 then D21 - D28
Oncovin	1.5 mg/m² /d (max 2mg/d)	D8, D15, D22 and D29
Imatinib	800 mg PO	J1 to J28
PL triple	Methotrexate 15 mg, Aracytine 40 mg, HC 15 mg	D1, D8 and D15
Neupogen	^{5} Hg/kg/d	up to PN >1000/mm3.

Assessment after induction treatment :

An informative post-induction myelogram should be performed on day 29 of this first course of treatment, with a 48-hour delay between the last injection of Neupogen and the performance of this myelogram, regardless of the platelet level.

-Control karyotype.

Evaluation of residual post-induction BCR-ABL disease must be carried out at this time, on the marrow, before starting the consolidation treatment (if BCR-M type transcript).

Consolidation cure :

Methotrexate	1000 mg/m² infused over 3 hours	J1, rescue with folinic acid
Aracytin	3000 mg/m² /12h, IV (over 2h)	J2 and J3
Imatinib	800 mg PO,	J1 to J14
PL	triples	J2
Neupogen	^{5} Hg/kg^j	D9 until PN >1000/mm3

Assessment of response after induction and consolidation :

A post-consolidation myelogram must be performed on day 21 of the consolidation cure, as soon as the PNN count > 1000/mm3 and the platelet count > 100,000/mm3, always allowing 48 hours between the last injection of Neupogen and the performance of this myelogram.

-Cytogenetic evaluation.

Evaluation of residual disease on marrow if M-BCR type transcribed.

If age < 50 and HLA-matched donor

Pre-transplant interphase: consists of 2 identical cycles combining Imatinib (at 600 mg/d), mëthotrexate and 6-mercaptopurine, as well as a triple LP, according to the following scheme:

Methotrexate	25 mg/m² PO	J1and J8
6-mercaptopurine	25 mg/m² , PO	D1 to D14 of each cycle
Imatinib	600 mg PO	J1 to J14
PL	triple	J1

Allogenic grafting : The conditioning will classically combine :

ICT: 10 Gy as a single dose with lung protection above 8 Gy or 12 Gy in 6 fractions with lung

protection above 8 or 10 Gy.
Cyclophosphamide: 60mg/kg on two consecutive days.
GVH prophylaxis: combination of cyclosporine A and methotrexate on D1, D3, D8 +/-D11.

Patients not eligible for allogeneic transplantation: Imatinib-Hyper CVAD interview		
Cures 3/5/7		
Vincristine	2 mg IVL	J11
Adriamycin	50 mg/m²	J4
Cyclophosphamide	300 mg/ m /12h²	J1, J2, J3
Dexamethasone	40 mg	D1 to D4 and D12 to D15
Imatinib	600 mg/d	J1 to J14
PL	triple	(cure 3 only)
NEUPOGEN	5 gg/kg/j	from D15.
Cures 4/6/8		
Methotrexate	1 g/m² in PIV over 3h	J1, rescue with 1 folinic acid
Aracytin	3 g/m /12h²	J2, J3
Imatinib	600 mg/d	J1 to J14
PL	triple	
NEUPOGEN	5 Pg/ kg/j	from J9 to PN >1000/mm .³
Maintenance		

Imatinib 600mg/d PO, daily, with monthly VCR-PND reinduction:
Vincristine 2mg IV once/month, D1; Prednisone 200mg/d once/month, D1 to D15.
At months 6 and 13, this treatment was replaced by two new courses of hyper CVAD lmatinib, identical to courses 6/8 (at month 13).
bcr-abl (if m BCR) or quantitative (if M BCR)/ 3 months.

-Radiotherapy of the encephalon :
*18Gy up to C2 at the start of maintenance treatment, on purinethol 25g/m2/d without MTX, CBC checked once a week.
*Radiation field: 2 lateral fields, facial mass (eye protection), base of skull+C1+C2.
-Curative meninge treatment :
Triple LPs: twice a week until normalisation, then according to protocol
Radiotherapy of the encephalon :
*if no indication for allogeneic transplantation: 24 Gy in 10 sessions up to C2, 5 sessions per week, at the start of maintenance treatment, under purinethol without MTX, CBC check 1x/week.
*If an allograft is indicated, this irradiation is carried out before the allograft at a dose of 15Gy in 10 sessions, 5 sessions per week + purinethol 25 mg/m2/d per os.

Appendix 4: WHO classification of haematological toxicity.

Toxicity	Grade 0	Grade 1	Grade 2	Grade]	Grade 4
Hemoglobins (Hb| W=13iflj/d	>11	<LIN-10,0g/dL	<10.0-11.0 d/<fl	<8.0-6.5g/dL	<6.5g/dL
Leukocytes VN=4DOOal0OOO	>4000	< LIN - 3000 / mm^{1}	< И ■ 2000 /mm^{1}	<2000-1000/mm^{1}	< 1000 /mm^{3}
Neutrophil Polynuclei VN="	>2000	< LIN- 1500 /mm^{1}	< 1500-1000 /mm^{1}	< 1000 - 500 /mm^{1}	< 500 / mm^{1}
Inserts VN = 15,000 to 400,000	> 100 000	<UN-75000/mm3	<75,000 - 50,000/mm3	< 50,000 - 25,000/mm]	<25,000/ mm]
Bleeding	Absences	Petechies	Moderate	Averages	Important
LIN: Lower Limit to Normal					

Appendix 5: Diagram of our study.

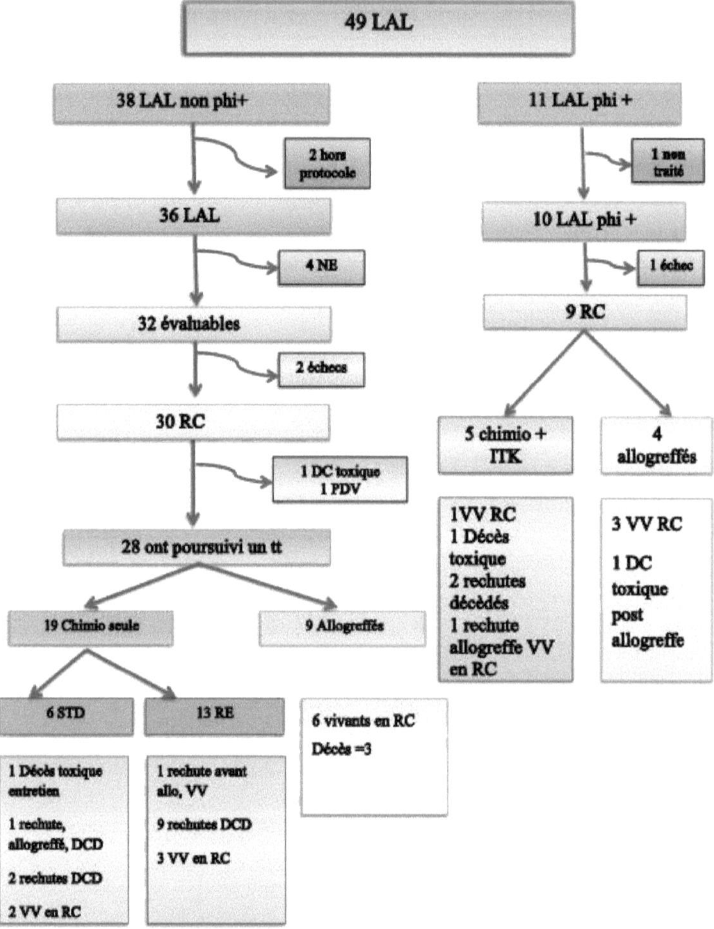

SUMMARY

Problem: Significant progress has been made in the treatment of ALL in children. However, results in adults are still unsatisfactory. The adaptation of current protocols to prognostic factors has improved therapeutic results. However, our results are less encouraging.

Aim of the study: The aim of this study is to evaluate the results of the GRAALL and GRAAPH protocols in the treatment of adult ALL and to propose a stratification and therapeutic algorithm adapted to the prognostic factors valid in our patients.

Methods: Our study is retrospective. It included adults followed for ALL diagnosed between January 2004 and December 2015 and treated according to the GRAALL and GRAAPH protocols at the Hematology Department of the Hedi Chaker University Hospital in Sfax.

We studied the diagnostic characteristics, therapeutic results, evolution and prognostic factors of our population.

Results and Discussion: We enrolled 49 patients, with a sex ratio of 0.88. The median age was 42 years, with 55% of our patients aged over 40 years. Hyperleukocytosis >30 G/l was observed in 28% of cases. In 65% of cases the patients were ALL-B, in 33% ALL-T and in 2% biphenotypic. Karyotyping was conclusive in 70% of cases, 51% of which had cytogenetic abnormalities. Corticoresistance and chemoresistance were observed in 11% and 17% of cases retrospectively. The overall CR rate was 93% for non-phi+ ALL and 90% for phi+ ALL, with failure rates of 5% and 10% respectively. 50% of our non-phi+ ALL patients relapsed during follow-up compared with 33% of our phi+ ALL patients. Allogeneic bone marrow transplantation significantly improved OS, ESRD and RFS in non-phi+ patients.

Conclusion: Adaptation of therapy certainly requires consideration of residual disease, introduction of Rituximab, intensification for high-risk cases and, why not, for phi+ ALL with allogeneic indications and no compatible donor, introduction of bone marrow autotransplantation, which will soon be practised in our department.

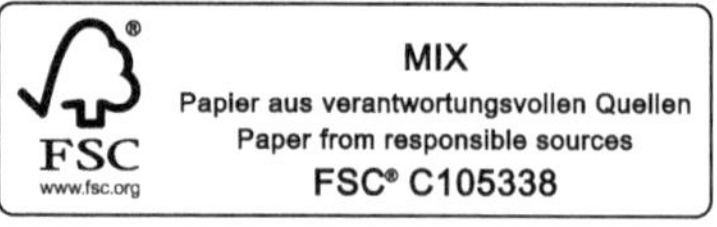

Printed by Books on Demand GmbH, Norderstedt / Germany